Keto Diet Cookbook for Beginners

500 Simple and Healthy Ketogenic Recipes That Will Make Your Life Insanely Easy

Dave Pine

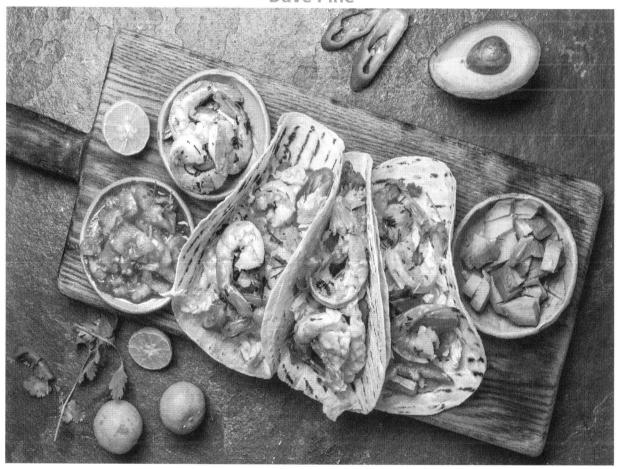

2019

Table Of Contents

Introduction

Do you want to make a change in your life? Do you want to become a healthier person who can enjoy a new and improved life? Then, you are definitely in the right place. You are about to discover a wonderful and very healthy diet that has changed millions of lives. We are talking about the Ketogenic diet, a lifestyle that will mesmerize you and that will make you a new person in no time.
So, let's sit back, relax and find out more about the Ketogenic diet.

A keto diet is a low carb one. This is the first and one of the most important things you should now. During such a diet, your body makes ketones in your liver and these are used as energy.
Your body will produce less insulin and glucose and a state of ketosis is induced.
Ketosis is a natural process that appears when our food intake is lower than usual. The body will soon adapt to this state and therefore you will be able to lose weight in no time but you will also become healthier and your physical and mental performances will improve.
But wait! These is not all! Your blood sugar levels will improve and you won't be predisposed to diabetes.
Also, epilepsy and heart diseases can be prevented if you are on a Ketogenic diet.
Your cholesterol will improve and you will feel amazing in no time.
How does that sound?

A Ketogenic diet is simple and easy to follow as long as you follow some simple rules.
You don't need to make huge changes but there are some things you should know.
So, here goes!

If you are on a Ketogenic diet you can't eat:
- Grains like corn, cereals, rice, etc
- Fruits like bananas
- Sugar
- Dry beans
- Honey
- Potatoes
- Yams

If you are on a Ketogenic diet you can eat:
- Greens like spinach, green beans, kale, bok choy, etc
- Meat like poultry, fish, pork, lamb, beef, etc
- Eggs
- Above ground veggies like cauliflower or broccoli, napa cabbage or regular cabbage
- Nuts and seeds
- Cheese
- Ghee or butter
- Avocados and all kind of berries
- Sweeteners like erythritol, splenda, stevia and others that contain only a few carbs

- Coconut oil
- Avocado oil
- Olive oil

The list of foods you are allowed to eat during a keto diet is permissive and rich as you can see for yourself.
So, we think it should be pretty easy for you to start such a diet.

If you've made this choice already, then, it's time you checked our amazing keto recipe collection.
You will discover 500 of the best Ketogenic recipes in the world and you will soon be able to make each and every one of these recipes.

Now let's start our magical culinary journey!
Ketogenic lifestyle…here we come!

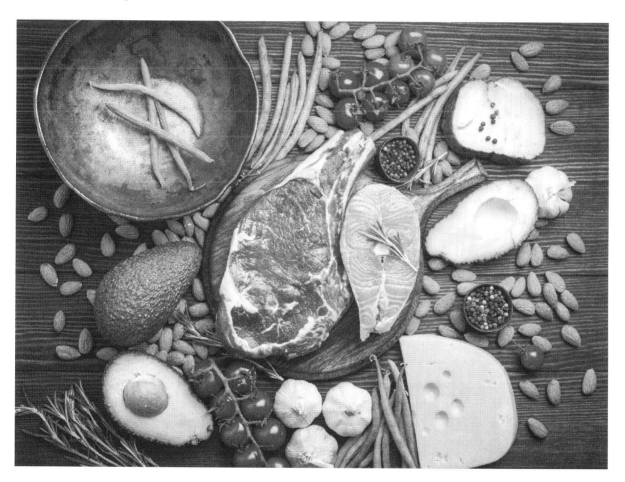

Ketogenic Recipes for Breakfast

Chili Tomatoes and Eggs
This recipe is perfect for breakfast!

Preparation time: 10 minutes
Cooking time: 20 minutes
Servings: 4

Ingredients:

- 1 tablespoon ghee, melted
- 2 shallots, chopped
- 2 chili peppers, minced
- Salt and black pepper to the taste
- 4 tomatoes, cubed
- 4 eggs, whisked
- 1 teaspoon sweet paprika
- 1 tablespoon chives, chopped

Directions:
Heat up a pan with the ghee over medium heat, add the shallots and the chili peppers, toss and sauté for 5 minutes. Add the tomatoes and the other ingredients except the eggs, toss and cook everything for 5 minutes more. Add the eggs, toss a bit, cook the mix for another 5 minutes, divide between plates and serve.

Nutrition: calories 119, fat 7.9, fiber 1.8, carbs 6.5, protein 6.9

Mushroom Omelet
You will feel full of energy all day with this keto breakfast!

Preparation time: 10 minutes
Cooking time: 20 minutes
Servings: 4

Ingredients:

- 2 spring onions, chopped
- ½ pound white mushrooms
- Salt and black pepper to the taste
- 4 eggs, whisked
- 1 tablespoon olive oil
- ½ teaspoon cumin, ground
- 1 tablespoon cilantro, chopped

Directions:
Heat up a pan with the oil over medium heat, add the spring onions and the mushrooms, toss and sauté for 5 minutes. Add the eggs and the rest of the ingredients, toss gently, spread into the pan, cover it and cook over medium heat for 15 minutes. Slice the omelet, divide it between plates and serve for breakfast.

Nutrition: calories 109, fat 8.1, fiber 0.8, carbs 2.9, protein 7.5

Bell Peppers and Avocado Bowls
Try a different keto breakfast each day!

Preparation time: 10 minutes
Cooking time: 15 minutes
Servings: 4

Ingredients:
- 2 tablespoons olive oil
- 2 shallots, chopped
- 1 red bell pepper, cut into strips
- 1 yellow bell pepper, cut into strips
- 1 green bell pepper, cut into strips
- 1 big avocado, peeled, pitted and cut into wedges
- 1 teaspoon sweet paprika
- ½ cup vegetable stock
- Salt and black pepper to the taste
- 1 tablespoon chives, chopped

Directions:
Heat up a pan with the oil medium heat, add the shallots and sauté them for 2 minutes. Add the bell peppers, avocado and the other ingredients except the chives, toss, bring to a simmer and cook over medium heat for 13 minutes more. Add the chives, toss, divide into bowls and serve for breakfast.

Nutrition: calories 194, fat 17.1, fiber 4.9, carbs 11.5, protein 2

Spinach and Eggs Salad
This taste delicious!

Preparation time: 5 minutes
Cooking time: 0 minutes
Servings: 4

Ingredients:
- 2 cups baby spinach
- 1 cup cherry tomatoes, cubed
- 1 tablespoon chives, chopped
- 4 eggs, hard boiled, peeled and roughly cubed
- Salt and black pepper to the taste
- 1 tablespoon lime juice
- 1 tablespoon olive oil

Directions:
In a bowl, combine the spinach with the tomatoes and the other ingredients, toss and serve for breakfast right away.

Nutrition: calories 107, fat 8, fiber 0.9, carbs 3.6, protein 6.4

Creamy Eggs
It's so tasty!

Preparation time: 10 minutes
Cooking time: 15 minutes
Servings: 4

Ingredients:
- 8 eggs, whisked
- 2 spring onions, chopped
- 1 tablespoon olive oil
- ½ cup heavy cream
- Salt and black pepper to the taste
- ½ cup mozzarella, shredded
- 1 tablespoon chives, chopped

Directions:
Heat up a pan with the oil over medium heat, add the spring onions, toss and sauté them for 3 minutes. Add the eggs mixed with the cream, salt and pepper and stir into the pan. Sprinkle the mozzarella, on top, cook the mix for 12 minutes, divide it between plates, sprinkle the chives on top and serve.

Nutrition: calories 220, fat 18.5, fiber 0.2, carbs 1.8, protein 12.5

Shrimp and Eggs Mix
It will surprise you with its taste!

Preparation time: 5 minutes
Cooking time: 11 minutes
Servings: 4

Ingredients:
- 8 eggs, whisked
- 1 tablespoon olive oil
- ½ pound shrimp, peeled, deveined and roughly chopped
- ¼ cup green onions, chopped
- 1 teaspoon sweet paprika
- Salt and black pepper to the taste
- 1 tablespoon cilantro, chopped

Directions:
Heat up a pan with the oil over medium heat, add the spring onions, toss and sauté for 2 minutes. Add the shrimp, stir and cook for 4 minutes more. Add the eggs, paprika, salt and pepper, toss and cook for 5 minutes more. Divide the mix between plates, sprinkle the cilantro on top and serve for breakfast.

Nutrition: calories 227, fat 13.3, fiber 0.4, carbs 2.3, protein 24.2

Garlicky Beef Bowls
These elements combine very well!

Preparation time: 10 minutes
Cooking time: 20 minutes
Servings: 4

Ingredients:

- 1 pound beef, ground
- 2 shallots, chopped
- 2 tablespoons tomato passata
- 1 green bell pepper, cut into strips
- 1 cup cherry tomatoes, halved
- 1 cup black olives, pitted and halved
- 1 tablespoon olive oil
- 2 green onions, chopped
- 3 garlic cloves, minced
- Salt and black pepper to the taste
- ½ tablespoon chives, chopped

Directions:

Heat up a pan with the oil over medium heat, add the shallots, toss and cook for 2 minutes. Add the beef, toss and brown it for 5 minutes more. Add the green bell pepper and the other ingredients, toss, cook over medium heat for 12 minutes more, divide into bowls and serve for breakfast.

Nutrition: calories 319, fat 14.4, fiber 3.3, carbs 10.3, protein 36.8

Tomato and Eggs Salad
This is truly the best keto breakfast salad!

Preparation time: 5 minutes
Cooking time: 0 minutes
Servings: 4

Ingredients:

- 4 eggs, hard boiled, peeled and cut into wedges
- 2 cups cherry tomatoes, halved
- 1 cup kalamata olives, pitted and halved
- 1 cup baby arugula
- 2 spring onions, chopped
- A pinch of salt and black pepper
- 1 tablespoon avocado oil

Directions:

In a salad bowl, combine the tomatoes with the eggs and the other ingredients, toss, divide into smaller bowls and serve for breakfast.

Nutrition: calories 126, fat 8.6, fiber 2.6, carbs 6.9, protein 6.9

Avocado Spread
This is so creamy!

Preparation time: 10 minutes
Cooking time: 0 minutes
Servings: 4

Ingredients:
- 2 avocados, peeled, pitted and chopped
- 1 tablespoon olive oil
- 1 tablespoon shallots, minced
- 1 tablespoon lime juice
- 1 tablespoon heavy cream
- Salt and black pepper to the taste
- 1 tablespoon chives, chopped

Directions:
In a blender, combine the avocado flesh with the oil, shallots and the other ingredients except the chives, pulse well, divide into bowls, sprinkle the chives on top and serve as a morning spread.

Nutrition: calories 253, fat 24.5, fiber 6.8, carbs 10.1, protein 2.1

Shrimp and Olives Pan
This is a perfect breakfast idea!

Preparation time: 10 minutes
Cooking time: 10 minutes
Servings: 4

Ingredients:
- 1 pound shrimp, peeled and deveined
- 1 cup black olives, pitted and halved
- ½ cup kalamata olives, pitted and halved
- 2 spring onions, chopped
- 2 teaspoons sweet paprika
- 1 tablespoon olive oil
- Salt and black pepper to the taste
- ½ cup heavy cream

Directions:
Heat up a pan with the oil over medium heat, add the onions, toss and cook for 2 minutes. Add the shrimp and the other ingredients except the cream, toss and cook for 4 minutes more. Add the cream, toss, cook over medium heat for another 4 minutes, divide everything between plates and serve for breakfast.

Nutrition: calories 263, fat 14.8, fiber 1.7, carbs 5.5, protein 26.7

Pork and Avocado Mix

Try a different breakfast today!

Preparation time: 10 minutes
Cooking time: 22 minutes
Servings: 4

Ingredients:

- ½ cup tomato passata
- 1 pound pork, ground
- 1 avocado, peeled, pitted and roughly cubed
- 1 tomato, cubed
- Salt and black pepper to the taste
- 8 eggs, whisked
- 2 spring onions, chopped
- 1 tablespoon avocado oil
- ½ teaspoon cayenne pepper
- 1 tablespoon chives, chopped

Directions:

Heat up a pan with the oil over medium heat, add the spring onions, stir and cook for 2 minutes. Add the meat, tomato and the cayenne pepper, toss and brown for 5 minutes more. Add the tomato passata, the avocado, eggs, salt and pepper, toss, cook over medium heat for 15 minutes more, divide into bowls and serve for breakfast.

Nutrition: calories 431, fat 26.1, fiber 4.1, carbs 6.8, protein 42.3

Beef Meatloaf

Pay attention and learn how to make this great breakfast in no time!

Preparation time: 10 minutes
Cooking time: 45 minutes
Servings: 6

Ingredients:

- 2 shallots, chopped
- 1 tablespoon olive oil
- 1 green bell pepper, chopped
- 2 garlic cloves, minced
- 2 eggs, whisked
- 1 pound beef, ground
- Salt and black pepper to the taste
- 1 tablespoon cilantro, chopped

Directions:

Heat up a pan with the oil over medium heat, add the shallots and the garlic, stir and cook for 5 minutes. In a bowl, combine the shallots and garlic with the meat and the other ingredients, stir well, shape your meatloaf and put it in a loaf pan. Introduce in the oven and cook at 380 degrees F for 40 minutes. Cool the meatloaf, divide between plates and serve for breakfast.

Nutrition: calories 192, fat 8.6, fiber 0.3, carbs 2.5, protein 25.1

Chili Spinach and Beef Mix
We recommend you try this keto breakfast as soon as possible!

Preparation time: 10 minutes
Cooking time: 26 minutes
Servings: 4

Ingredients:

- 1 pound beef meat, ground
- 1 tablespoons avocado oil
- 2 shallots, chopped
- 2 garlic cloves, minced
- 2 teaspoons red chili flakes
- 1 tablespoon tomato passata
- 1 cup baby spinach
- 1 teaspoon chili powder
- Salt and black pepper to the taste

Directions:

Heat up a pan with the oil over medium heat, add the shallots and the garlic, stir and cook for 3 minutes.
Add the meat and brown it for 5 minutes.
Add the chili flakes and the other ingredients, toss, cook over medium heat for 15 minutes, divide into bowls and serve for breakfast.

Nutrition: calories 239, fat 9.2, fiber 1.1, carbs 3.2, protein 34.1

Zucchini Spread
It's going to be so tasty!

Preparation time: 10 minutes
Cooking time: 17 minutes
Servings: 4

Ingredients:

- 1 pound zucchinis, roughly cubed
- 1 cup heavy cream
- 2 shallots, chopped
- 1 tablespoon lime juice
- 1 tablespoon avocado oil
- Salt and black pepper to the taste
- 1 tablespoon basil, chopped

Directions:

Heat up a pan with the oil over medium high heat, add the shallots, stir and sauté for 2 minutes. Add the zucchinis and the other ingredients, stir, cook over medium heat for 15 minutes, cool down, transfer to a blender, pulse a few times, divide into bowls and serve as a morning spread.

Nutrition: calories 240, fat 7.6, fiber 2, carbs 5.9, protein 11.2

Spinach Omelet
You've got to try this!

Preparation time: 10 minutes
Cooking time: 20 minutes
Servings: 4

Ingredients:
- 8 eggs, whisked
- 1 cup baby spinach
- A pinch of salt and black pepper
- 1 tablespoon olive oil
- 2 spring onions, chopped
- 1 teaspoon sweet paprika
- 1 teaspoon cumin, ground
- 1 tablespoon chives, chopped

Directions:
Heat up a pan with the oil over medium heat, add the spring onions, paprika and cumin, stir and sauté for 5 minutes. Add the eggs, the spinach, salt and pepper, toss, spread into the pan, cover it and cook for 15 minutes. prinkle the chives on top, divide everything between plates and serve.

Nutrition: calories 345, fat 12, fiber 1.5, carbs 8, protein 13.3

Sage Zucchini Cakes
This is incredibly tasty and easy to make for breakfast!

Preparation time: 10 minutes
Cooking time: 12 minutes
Servings: 4

Ingredients:
- 1 pound zucchinis, grated and excess water drained
- Salt and black pepper to the taste
- 1 tablespoon almond flour
- 1 egg, whisked
- 1 tablespoon sage, chopped
- 2 tablespoons olive oil

Directions:
In a bowl, combine the zucchinis with the flour and the other ingredients except the oil, stir well and shape medium cakes out of this mix. Heat up a pan with the oil over medium heat, add the cakes, cook them for 5-6 minutes on each side, drain excess grease on paper towels, divide the cakes between plates and serve for breakfast.

Nutrition: calories 320, fat 13.32, fiber 5.2, carbs 10, protein 12.1

Pork Casserole

It's so amazing! You must make it for breakfast tomorrow!

Preparation time: 10 minutes
Cooking time: 45 minutes
Servings: 4

Ingredients:

- 1 pound pork, ground
- Salt and black pepper to the taste
- 2 shallots, chopped
- 2 garlic cloves, minced
- 1 tablespoon olive oil
- 2 red bell peppers, roughly cubed
- 2 tomatoes, cubed
- 1 cup mozzarella, shredded
- 2 tablespoons parsley, chopped

Directions:

Heat up a pan with the oil over medium heat, add the shallots and the garlic and sauté for 5 minutes. Add the meat, bell peppers and the tomatoes, stir and cook for 5 minutes more. Spread this into a casserole, sprinkle the mozzarella and the parsley on top, introduce in the oven and cook at 380 degrees F for 35 minutes. Divide the mix between plates and serve for breakfast.

Nutrition: calories 340, fat 28, fiber 5.3, carbs 6.3, protein 17.6

Leeks and Eggs Mix

Preparation time: 5 minutes
Cooking time: 15 minutes
Servings: 4

Ingredients:

- 3 leeks, sliced
- 8 eggs, whisked
- 1 tablespoon avocado oil
- ¼ cup almond milk
- Salt and black pepper to the taste
- ¼ teaspoon garlic powder
- 1 teaspoon sweet paprika
- 1 tablespoon cilantro, chopped

Directions:

Heat up a pan with the oil over medium heat, add the leeks, garlic powder and the paprika, stir and sauté for 5 minutes. Add the eggs mixed with the milk, salt and pepper, stir, cook for 10 minutes more, divide between plates, sprinkle the cilantro on top and serve.

Nutrition: calories 340, fat 12, fiber 3.2, carbs 8, protein 23

Broccoli and Eggs Salad

Preparation time: 10 minutes
Cooking time: 0 minutes
Servings: 4

Ingredients:
- 1 pound broccoli florets, steamed
- 4 eggs, hard boiled, peeled and cut into wedges
- 2 spring onions, chopped
- ½ teaspoon chili powder
- 1 tablespoon olive oil
- 1 tablespoon lime juice
- Salt and black pepper to the taste

Directions:
In a bowl, combine the broccoli with the eggs and the other ingredients, toss and serve for breakfast.

Nutrition: calories 250, fat 11.2, fiber 4, carbs 5.6, protein 6.20

Zucchini Casserole
Try this Ketogenic breakfast today!

Preparation time: 10 minutes
Cooking time: 35 minutes
Servings: 4

Ingredients:
- 1 pound zucchinis, roughly cubed
- 1 cup mozzarella, shredded
- 1 shallot, chopped
- 1 tablespoon avocado oil
- 1 cup cherry tomatoes, chopped
- 4 eggs, whisked
- 1 tablespoon cilantro, chopped
- Salt and black pepper to the taste
- ½ cup kalamata olives, pitted and sliced

Directions:
Heat up a pan with the oil over medium heat, add the shallot and the zucchinis and cook for 3 minutes. Add the tomatoes, olives, salt and pepper, stir and cook for 2 minutes more. Pour the eggs mixed with the cheese and the cilantro on top, spread over the zucchinis mix, introduce in the oven and bake at 380 degrees F for 30 minutes. Cool the casserole down, slice and serve.

Nutrition: calories 135, fat 8.1, fiber 2.5, carbs 7.8, protein 9.5

Creamy Walnuts Bowls

This is just delicious!

Preparation time: 5 minutes
Cooking time: 10 minutes
Servings: 2
Ingredients:

- 1 teaspoon nutmeg, ground
- 1 and ½ cups walnuts
- 1 teaspoon stevia
- 1 teaspoon vanilla extract
- ¾ cup coconut cream

Directions:

Heat up a pan over medium heat, add the walnuts, nutmeg and the other ingredients, toss, cook for 10 minutes, divide into bowls and serve.

Nutrition: calories 200, fat 12, fiber 4, carbs 8, protein 4.5

Coconut Berries Bowls

A Ketogenic berries breakfast salad is the best idea ever!

Preparation time: 5 minutes
Cooking time: 0 minutes
Servings: 4
Ingredients:

- 1 cup blackberries
- 1 cup strawberries
- 1 cup raspberries
- 1 tablespoon lime juice
- ¼ cup almonds, cubed
- 2 teaspoons coconut oil, melted

Directions:

In a bowl, combine the strawberries with the blackberries and the rest of the ingredients, toss, divide into small bowls and serve for breakfast.

Nutrition: calories 200, fat 7.5, fiber 4, carbs 5.7, protein 8

Chia Bowls

It's a great way to start your day!

Preparation time: 10 minutes
Cooking time: 0 minutes.
Servings: 2
Ingredients:

- ¼ cup walnuts, chopped
- 1 and ½ cups almond milk
- 2 tablespoons chia seeds
- 1 tablespoon stevia
- 1 teaspoon vanilla extract

Directions:

In a bowl, combine the almond milk with the chia seeds and the rest of the ingredients, toss, leave the mix aside for 10 minutes and serve for breakfast.

Nutrition: calories 200, fat 8.3, fiber 2, carbs 5, protein 4

Tomato and Avocado Salad
You will be surprised! It's amazing!

Preparation time: 5 minutes
Cooking time: 0 minutes
Servings: 4

Ingredients:
- 2 cups cherry tomatoes, halved
- 2 avocados, pitted, peeled and cut into wedges
- A pinch of salt and black pepper
- 1 tablespoon olive oil
- 1 cucumber, sliced
- ½ cup kalamata olives, pitted and halved
- 1 tablespoon lime juice

Directions:
In a bowl, combine the tomatoes with the avocados and the other ingredients, toss and serve for breakfast.

Nutrition: calories 400, fat 9.2, fiber 4, carbs 5.5, protein 13.2

Salmon Cakes
This is a Ketogenic breakfast idea you should try soon!

Preparation time: 5 minutes
Cooking time: 10 minutes
Servings: 4

Ingredients:
- 1 pound salmon fillets, boneless, skinless and minced
- 1 egg, whisked
- 2 spring onions, chopped
- 1 tablespoon cilantro, chopped
- 2 tablespoons almond flour
- A pinch of salt and black pepper
- 2 tablespoons olive oil

Directions:
In a bowl, mix the salmon with the egg and the other ingredients except the oil, stir well and shape medium cakes out of this mix. Heat up a pan with the oil over medium heat, add the salmon cakes, cook them for 5 minutes on each side, divide between plates and serve for breakfast.

Nutrition: calories 249, fat 16.8, fiber 0.6, carbs 1.4, protein 24.3

Kale Frittata
These will really make your day much easier!

Preparation time: 10 minutes
Cooking time: 30 minutes
Servings: 4

Ingredients:
- 8 eggs, whisked
- 2 shallots, chopped
- 1 tablespoon avocado oil
- 1 cup kale, torn
- Salt and black pepper to the taste
- ¼ cup mozzarella, shredded
- 2 tablespoons chives, chopped

Directions:
Heat up a pan with the oil over medium heat, add the shallots, stir and cook for 5 minutes. Add the kale, stir and cook for 4 minutes more. Add the eggs mixed with the mozzarella, spread into the pan, sprinkle the chives on top and bake at 390 degrees F for 20 minutes. Divide the frittata between plates and serve.

Nutrition: calories 140, fat 6.7, fiber 1, carbs 4.3, protein 10

Spinach and Cauliflower Pan
It's a Ketogenic breakfast full of nutrients!

Preparation time: 10 minutes
Cooking time: 18 minutes
Servings: 4

Ingredients:
- 1 pound cauliflower florets
- 1 cup baby spinach
- 2 shallots, chopped
- 1 tablespoon olive oil
- 1 tablespoon balsamic vinegar
- 1 tablespoon parsley, chopped
- ½ cup walnuts, roughly chopped
- Salt and black pepper to the taste

Directions:
Heat up a pan with the oil over medium heat, add the shallots, stir and cook for 3 minutes. Add the cauliflower and the rest of the ingredients, toss, cook over medium heat for 15 minutes more, divide into bowls and serve for breakfast.

Nutrition: calories 140, fat 9.3, fiber 3, carbs 4, protein 8

Cauliflower Omelet
It's a tasty Ketogenic omelet!

Preparation time: 10 minutes
Cooking time: 15 minutes
Servings: 4

Ingredients:
- 4 eggs, whisked
- 1 cup cauliflower florets, chopped
- 2 spring onions, chopped
- 1 tablespoon olive oil
- ½ cup heavy cream
- ½ teaspoon sweet paprika
- Salt and black pepper to the taste
- 1 tablespoon chives, chopped

Directions:
Heat up a pan with the oil over medium heat, add the onion and the cauliflower, stir and sauté for 5 minutes. Add the eggs mixed with the cream, paprika, salt and pepper, toss, spread into the pan, cook over medium heat for 10 minutes, divide between plates, sprinkle the chives on top and serve.

Nutrition: calories 200, fat 4, fiber 6, carbs 5, protein 10

Chicken Casserole
It's a savory Ketogenic breakfast you can try today!

Preparation time: 10 minutes
Cooking time: 45 minutes
Servings: 4

Ingredients:
- 1 pound chicken breast, boneless, skinless and ground
- 2 shallots, chopped
- 1 tablespoon coconut oil, melted
- 1 cup baby spinach
- 4 eggs, whisked
- ½ cup parmesan, grated
- Salt and black pepper to the taste
- ½ teaspoon garlic powder

Directions:
Heat up a pan with the oil over medium heat, add the shallots, stir and cook for 5 minutes. Add the meat and brown for 5 minutes more. Add the eggs mixed with the garlic and toss. Sprinkle the parmesan on top, introduce in the oven and bake at 390 degrees F for 35 minutes. Divide the mix between plates and serve.

Nutrition: calories 273, fat 13.7, fiber 0.2, carbs 2.2, protein 34.5

Spiced Eggs
Try this healthy keto breakfast really soon!

Preparation time: 10 minutes
Cooking time: 15 minutes
Servings: 4

Ingredients:
- 1 tablespoon avocado oil
- 2 spring onions, chopped
- 1 tablespoon cilantro, chopped
- 4 eggs, whisked
- 1 teaspoon cumin, ground
- 1 teaspoon allspice, ground
- 1 teaspoon nutmeg, ground
- Salt and black pepper to the taste
- 1 tablespoons parsley, chopped

Directions:
Heat up a pan with the oil over medium heat, add the spring onions, stir and cook for 2 minutes. Add the eggs and the other ingredients, stir, spread into the pan and cook over medium heat for 13 minutes. Divide the eggs between plates and serve for breakfast.

Nutrition: calories 140, fat 6, fiber 2, carbs 10, protein 12

Avocado Muffins
If you like avocado recipes, then you should really try this next one soon!

Preparation time: 10 minutes
Cooking time: 20 minutes
Servings: 12

Ingredients:
- 4 eggs
- 6 bacon slices, chopped
- 1 yellow onion, chopped
- 1 cup coconut milk
- 2 cups avocado, pitted, peeled and chopped
- Salt and black pepper to the taste
- ½ teaspoon baking soda
- ½ cup coconut flour

Directions:
Heat up a pan over medium heat, add onion and bacon, stir and brown for a few minutes. In a bowl, mash avocado pieces with a fork and whisk well with the eggs. Add milk, salt, pepper, baking soda and coconut flour and stir everything. Add bacon mix and stir again. Grease a muffin tray with the coconut oil, divide eggs and avocado mix into the tray, introduce in the oven at 350 degrees F and bake for 20 minutes. Divide muffins on plates and serve them for breakfast.

Nutrition: calories 200, fat 7, fiber 4, carbs 7, protein 5

Bacon And Lemon Breakfast Muffins

We are sure you've never tried something like this before! It's a perfect keto breakfast!

Preparation time: 10 minutes
Cooking time: 20 minutes
Servings: 12

Ingredients:

- 1 cup bacon, finely chopped
- Salt and black pepper to the taste
- ½ cup ghee, melted
- 3 cups almond flour
- 1 teaspoon baking soda
- 4 eggs
- 2 teaspoons lemon thyme

Directions:

In a bowl, mix flour with baking soda and eggs and stir well. Add ghee, lemon thyme, bacon, salt and pepper and whisk well. Divide this into a lined muffin pan, introduce in the oven at 350 degrees F and bake for 20 minutes. Leave muffins to cool down a bit, divide on plates and serve them.

Nutrition: calories 213, fat 7, fiber 2, carbs 9, protein 8

Cheese And Oregano Muffins

We will make you love keto muffins from now on!

Preparation time: 10 minutes
Cooking time: 25 minutes
Servings: 6

Ingredients:

- 2 tablespoons olive oil
- 1 egg
- 2 tablespoons parmesan cheese
- ½ teaspoon oregano, dried
- 1 cup almond flour
- ¼ teaspoon baking soda
- Salt and black pepper to the taste
- ½ cup coconut milk
- 1 cup cheddar cheese, grated

Directions:

In a bowl, mix flour with oregano, salt, pepper, parmesan and baking soda and stir. In another bowl, mix coconut milk with egg and olive oil and stir well. Combine the 2 mixtures and whisk well. Add cheddar cheese, stir, pour this a lined muffin tray, introduce in the oven at 350 degrees F for 25 minutes. Leave your muffins to cool down for a few minutes, divide them on plates and serve.

Nutrition: calories 160, fat 3, fiber 2, carbs 6, protein 10

Delicious Turkey Breakfast
Try a Ketogenic turkey breakfast for a change!

Preparation time: 10 minutes
Cooking time: 20 minutes
Servings: 1

Ingredients:

- 2 avocado slices
- Salt and black pepper
- 2 bacon sliced
- 2 turkey breast slices, already cooked
- 2 tablespoons coconut oil
- 2 eggs, whisked

Directions:

Heat up a pan over medium heat, add bacon slices and brown them for a few minutes. Meanwhile, heat up another pan with the oil over medium heat, add eggs, salt and pepper and scramble them. Divide turkey breast slices on 2 plates. Divide scrambled eggs on each. Divide bacon slices and avocado slices as well and serve.

Nutrition: calories 135, fat 7, fiber 2, carbs 4, protein 10

Amazing Burrito
Can you have a burrito for breakfast? Of course, you can!

Preparation time: 10 minutes
Cooking time: 16 minutes
Servings: 1

Ingredients:

- 1 teaspoon coconut oil
- 1 teaspoon garlic powder
- 1 teaspoon cumin, ground
- ¼ pound beef meat, ground
- 1 teaspoon sweet paprika
- 1 teaspoon onion powder
- 1 small red onion, julienned
- 1 teaspoon cilantro, chopped
- Salt and black pepper to the taste
- 3 eggs

Directions:

Heat up a pan over medium heat, add beef and brown for a few minutes. Add salt, pepper, cumin, garlic and onion powder and paprika, stir, cook for 4 minutes more and take off heat. In a bowl, mix eggs with salt and pepper and whisk well. Heat up a pan with the oil over medium heat, add egg, spread evenly and cook for 6 minutes. Transfer your egg burrito to a plate, divide beef mix, add onion and cilantro, roll and serve.

Nutrition: calories 280, fat 12, fiber 4, carbs 7, protein 14

Amazing Breakfast Hash
This breakfast hash is just right for you!

Preparation time: 10 minutes
Cooking time: 16 minutes
Servings: 2

Ingredients:

- 1 tablespoon coconut oil
- 2 garlic cloves, minced
- ½ cup beef stock
- Salt and black pepper to the taste
- 1 yellow onion, chopped
- 2 cups corned beef, chopped
- 1 pound radishes, cut in quarters

Directions:
Heat up a pan with the oil over medium high heat, add onion, stir and cook for 4 minutes. Add radishes, stir and cook for 5 minutes. Add garlic, stir and cook for 1 minute more. Add stock, beef, salt and pepper, stir, cook for 5 minutes, take off heat and serve.

Nutrition: calories 240, fat 7, fiber 3, carbs 12, protein 8

Brussels Sprouts Delight
This is so tasty and very easy to make! It's a great keto breakfast idea for you!

Preparation time: 10 minutes
Cooking time: 12 minutes
Servings: 3

Ingredients:

- 3 eggs
- Salt and black pepper to the taste
- 1 tablespoon ghee, melted
- 2 shallots, minced
- 2 garlic cloves, minced
- 12 ounces Brussels sprouts, thinly sliced
- 2 ounces bacon, chopped
- 1 and ½ tablespoons apple cider vinegar

Directions:
Heat up a pan over medium heat, add bacon, stir, cook until it's crispy, transfer to a plate and leave aside for now. Heat up the pan again over medium heat, add shallots and garlic, stir and cook for 30 seconds. Add Brussels sprouts, salt, pepper and apple cider vinegar, stir and cook for 5 minutes. Return bacon to pan, stir and cook for 5 minutes more. Add ghee, stir and make a hole in the center. Crack eggs into the pan, cook until they are done and serve right away.

Nutrition: calories 240, fat 7, fiber 4, carbs 7, protein 12

Breakfast Cereal Nibs
Pay attention and learn how to prepare the best keto cereal nibs!

Preparation time: 10 minutes
Cooking time: 45minutes
Servings: 4

Ingredients:
- 4 tablespoons hemp hearts
- ½ cup chia seeds
- 1 cup water
- 1 tablespoon vanilla extract
- 1 tablespoon psyllium powder
- 2 tablespoons coconut oil
- 1 tablespoon swerve
- 2 tablespoons cocoa nibs

Directions:
In a bowl, mix chia seeds with water, stir and leave aside for 5 minutes. Add hemp hearts, vanilla extract, psyllium powder, oil and swerve and stir well with your mixer. Add cocoa nibs, and stir until you obtain a dough. Divide dough in 2 pieces, shape into cylinder form, place on a lined baking sheet, flatten well, cover with a parchment paper, introduce in the oven at 285 degrees F and bake for 20 minutes. Remove the parchment paper and bake for 25 minutes more. Take cylinders out of the oven, leave aside to cool down and cut into small pieces. Serve in the morning with some almond milk.

Nutrition: calories 245, fat 12, fiber 12, carbs 2, protein 9

Breakfast Chia Pudding
Try a chia pudding this morning!

Preparation time: 10 minutes
Cooking time: 30 minutes
Servings: 2

Ingredients:
- 2 tablespoons coffee
- 2 cups water
- 1/3 cup chia seeds
- 1 tablespoon swerve
- 1 tablespoon vanilla extract
- 2 tablespoons cocoa nibs
- 1/3 cup coconut cream

Directions:
Heat up a small pot with the water over medium heat, bring to a boil, add coffee, simmer for 15 minutes, take off heat and strain into a bowl. Add vanilla extract, coconut cream, swerve, cocoa nibs and chia seeds, stir well, keep in the fridge for 30 minutes, divide into 2 breakfast bowls and serve.

Nutrition: calories 100, fat 0.4, fiber 4, carbs 3, protein 3

Delicious Hemp Porridge
It's a hearty and 100% keto breakfast idea!

Preparation time: 3 minutes
Cooking time: 3 minutes
Servings: 1

Ingredients:
- 1 tablespoon chia seeds
- 1 cup almond milk
- 2 tablespoons flax seeds
- ½ cup hemp hearts
- ½ teaspoon cinnamon, round
- 1 tablespoon stevia
- ¾ teaspoon vanilla extract
- ¼ cup almond flour
- 1 tablespoon hemp hearts for serving

Directions:
In a pan, mix almond milk with ½ cup hemp hearts, chia seeds, stevia, flax seeds, cinnamon and vanilla extract, stir well and heat up over medium heat. Cook for 2 minutes, take off heat, add almond flour, stir well and pour into a bowl. Top with 1 tablespoon hemp hearts and serve.

Nutrition: calories 230, fat 12, fiber 7, carbs 3, protein 43

Simple Breakfast Cereal
It's so easy to make a tasty keto breakfast!

Preparation time: 10 minutes
Cooking time: 3 minutes
Servings: 2

Ingredients:
- ½ cup coconut, shredded
- 4 teaspoons ghee
- 2 cups almond milk
- 1 tablespoon stevia
- A pinch of salt
- 1/3 cup macadamia nuts, chopped
- 1/3 cup walnuts, chopped
- 1/3 cup flax seed

Directions:
Heat up a pot with the ghee over medium heat, add milk, coconut, salt, macadamia nuts, walnuts, flax seed and stevia and stir well. Cook for 3 minutes, stir again, take off heat and leave aside for 10 minutes. Divide into 2 bowls and serve.

Nutrition: calories 140, fat 3, fiber 2, carbs 1.5, protein 7

Simple Egg Porridge

It's so simple and tasty!

Preparation time: 10 minutes
Cooking time: 4 minutes
Servings: 2

Ingredients:

- 2 eggs
- 1 tablespoon stevia
- 1/3 cup heavy cream
- 2 tablespoons ghee, melted
- A pinch of cinnamon, ground

Directions:

In a bowl, mix eggs with stevia and heavy cream and whisk well. Heat up a pan with the ghee over medium high heat, add egg mix and cook until they are done. Transfer to 2 bowls, sprinkle cinnamon on top and serve.

Nutrition: calories 340, fat 12, fiber 10, carbs 3, protein 14

Delicious Pancakes

Why don't you try these delicious keto pancakes today?

Preparation time: 3 minutes
Cooking time: 12 minutes
Servings: 4

Ingredients:

- ½ teaspoon cinnamon, ground
- 1 teaspoon stevia
- 2 eggs
- Cooking spray
- 2 ounces cream cheese

Directions:

In your blender, mix eggs with cream cheese, stevia and cinnamon and blend well. Heat up a pan with some cooking spray over medium high heat, pour ¼ of the batter, spread well, cook for 2 minutes, flip and cook for 1 minute more. Transfer to a plate and repeat the action with the rest of the batter. Serve them right away.

Nutrition: calories 344, fat 23, fiber 12, carbs 3, protein 16

Almond Pancakes

These are so delicious! Try them!

Preparation time: 10 minutes
Cooking time: 10 minutes
Servings: 12

Ingredients:

- 6 eggs
- A pinch of salt
- ½ cup coconut flour
- ¼ cup stevia
- 1/3 cup coconut, shredded
- ½ teaspoon baking powder
- 1 cup almond milk
- ¼ cup coconut oil
- 1 teaspoon almond extract
- ¼ cup almonds, toasted
- 2 ounces cocoa chocolate
- Cooking spray

Directions:

In a bowl, mix coconut flour with stevia, salt, baking powder and coconut and stir. Add coconut oil, eggs, almond milk and the almond extract and stir well again. Add chocolate and almonds and whisk well again. Heat up a pan with cooking spray over medium heat, add 2 tablespoons batter, spread into a circle, cook until it's golden, flip, cook again until it's done and transfer to a pan. Repeat with the rest of the batter and serve your pancakes right away.

Nutrition: calories 266, fat 13, fiber 8, carbs 10, protein 11

Delicious Pumpkin Pancakes

These keto pumpkin pancakes will make your day!

Preparation time: 10 minutes
Cooking time: 15 minutes
Servings: 6

Ingredients:

- 1 ounce egg white protein
- 2 ounces hazelnut flour
- 2 ounces flax seeds, ground
- 1 teaspoon baking powder
- 1 cup coconut cream
- 1 tablespoon chai masala
- 1 teaspoon vanilla extract
- ½ cup pumpkin puree
- 3 eggs
- 5 drops stevia
- 1 tablespoon swerve
- 1 teaspoon coconut oil

Directions:

In a bowl, mix flax seeds with hazelnut flour, egg white protein, baking powder and chai masala and stir. In another bowl, mix coconut cream with vanilla extract, pumpkin puree, eggs, stevia and swerve and stir well. Combine the 2 mixtures and stir well. Heat up a pan with the oil over medium high heat, pour 1/6 of the batter, spread into a circle, cover, reduce heat to low, cook for 3 minutes on each side and transfer to a plate. Repeat with the rest of the batter and serve your pumpkin pancakes right away.

Nutrition: calories 400, fat 23, fiber 4, carbs 5, protein 21

Simple Breakfast French Toast

Believe it or not, this is a keto breakfast!

Preparation time: 5 minutes
Cooking time: 45 minutes
Servings: 18

Ingredients:

- 1 cup whey protein
- 12 egg whites
- 4 ounces cream cheese

For the French toast:

- 1 teaspoon vanilla
- ½ cup coconut milk

- 2 eggs
- 1 teaspoon cinnamon, ground
- ½ cup ghee, melted
- ½ cup almond milk
- ½ cup swerve

Directions:

In a bowl, mix 12 egg whites with your mixer for a few minutes. Add protein and stir gently. Add cream cheese and stir again. Pour this into 2 greased bread pans, introduce in the oven at 325 degrees F and bake for 45 minutes. Leave breads to cool down and slice them in 18 pieces. In a bowl, mix 2 eggs with vanilla, cinnamon and coconut milk and whisk well. Dip bread slices in this mix. Heat up a pan with some coconut oil over medium heat, add bread slices, cook until they are golden on each side and divide on plates. Heat up a pan with the ghee over high heat, add almond milk and heat up well. Add swerve, stir and take off heat. Leave aside to cool down a bit and drizzle over French toasts.

Nutrition: calories 200, fat 12, fiber 1, carbs 1, protein 7

Amazing Waffles

Get ready for a really tasty breakfast!

Preparation time: 10 minutes
Cooking time: 20 minutes
Servings: 5

Ingredients:

- 5 eggs, separated
- 3 tablespoons almond milk
- 1 teaspoon baking powder
- 3 tablespoons stevia

- 4 tablespoons coconut flour
- 2 teaspoon vanilla
- 4 ounces ghee, melted

Directions:

In a bowl, whisk egg white using your mixer. In another bowl mix flour with stevia, baking powder and egg yolks and whisk well. Add vanilla, ghee and milk and stir well again. Add egg white and stir gently everything. Pour some of the mix into your waffle makes and cook until it's golden. Repeat with the rest of the batter and serve your waffles right away.

Nutrition: calories 240, fat 23, fiber 2, carbs 4, protein 7

Baked Granola
This is so amazing and tasty! We love it!

Preparation time: 10 minutes
Cooking time: 60 minutes
Servings: 4

Ingredients:
- ½ cup almonds, chopped
- 1 cup pecans, chopped
- ½ cup walnuts, chopped
- ½ cup coconut, flaked
- ¼ cup flax meal
- ½ cup almond milk
- ¼ cup sunflower seeds
- ¼ cup pepitas
- ½ cup stevia
- ¼ cup ghee, melted
- 1 teaspoon honey
- 1 teaspoon vanilla
- 1 teaspoon cinnamon, ground
- A pinch of salt
- ½ teaspoon nutmeg
- ¼ cup water

Directions:
In a bowl, mix almonds with pecans, walnuts, coconut, flax meal, milk, sunflower seeds, pepitas, stevia, ghee, honey, vanilla, cinnamon, salt, nutmeg and water and whisk very well. Grease a baking sheet with parchment paper, spread granola mix and press well. Cover with another piece of parchment paper, introduce in the oven at 250 degrees F and bake for 1 hour. Take granola out of the oven, leave aside to cool down, break into pieces and serve.

Nutrition: calories 340, fat 32, fiber 12, carbs 20, protein 20

Amazing Smoothie
This smoothie is the best!

Preparation time: 5 minutes
Cooking time: 0 minutes
Servings: 1

Ingredients:
- 2 brazil nuts
- 1 cup coconut milk
- 10 almonds
- 2 cups spinach leaves
- 1 teaspoon green powder
- 1 teaspoon whey protein
- 1 tablespoon psyllium seeds
- 1 tablespoon potato starch

Directions:
In your blender, mix spinach with brazil nuts, coconut milk and almonds and blend well. Add green powder, whey protein, potato starch and psyllium seeds and blend well again. Pour into a tall glass and consume for breakfast.

Nutrition: calories 340, fat 30, fiber 7, carbs 7, protein 12

Refreshing Breakfast Smoothie
It's so healthy and fresh! We love it!

Preparation time: 5 minutes
Cooking time: 0 minutes
Servings: 6

Ingredients:
- 1 cup lettuce leaves
- 4 cups water
- 2 tablespoons parsley leaves
- 1 tablespoon ginger, grated
- 1 tablespoon swerve
- 1 cup cucumber, sliced
- ½ avocado, pitted and peeled
- ½ cup kiwi, peeled and sliced
- 1/3 cup pineapple, chopped

Directions:
In your blender, mix water with lettuce leaves, pineapple, parsley, cucumber, ginger, kiwi, avocado and swerve and blend very well. Pour into glasses and serve for a keto breakfast.

Nutrition: calories 60, fat 2, fiber 3, carbs 3, protein 1

Amazing Breakfast In A Glass
Don't bother making something complex for breakfast! Try this amazing keto drink!

Preparation time: 3 minutes
Cooking time: 0 minutes
Servings: 2

Ingredients:
- 10 ounces canned coconut milk
- 1 cup favorite greens
- ¼ cup cocoa nibs
- 1 cup water
- 1 cup cherries, frozen
- ¼ cup cocoa powder
- 1 small avocado, pitted and peeled
- ¼ teaspoon turmeric

Directions:
In your blender, mix coconut milk with avocado, cocoa powder, cherries and turmeric and blend well. Add water, greens and cocoa nibs, blend for 2 minutes more, pour into glasses and serve.

Nutrition: calories 100, fat 3, fiber 2, carbs 3, protein 5

Delicious Chicken Quiche
It's so delicious that you will ask for more!

Preparation time: 10 minutes
Cooking time: 45 minutes
Servings: 5

Ingredients:

- 7 eggs
- 2 cups almond flour
- 2 tablespoons coconut oil
- Salt and black pepper to the taste
- 2 zucchinis, grated
- ½ cup heavy cream
- 1 teaspoon fennel seeds
- 1 teaspoon oregano, dried
- 1 pound chicken meat, ground

Directions:

In your food processor, blend almond flour with a pinch of salt. Add 1 egg and coconut oil and blend well Place dough in a greased pie pan and press well on the bottom. Heat up a pan over medium heat, add chicken meat, brown for a couple of minutes, take off heat and leave aside. In a bowl, mix 6 eggs with salt, pepper, oregano, cream and fennel seeds and whisk well. Add chicken meat and stir again. Pour this into pie crust, spread, introduce in the oven at 350 degrees F and bake for 40 minutes. Leave pie to cool down a bit before slicing and serving it for breakfast!

Nutrition: calories 300, fat 23, fiber 3, carbs 4, protein 18

Delicious Steak And Eggs
This is so rich and hearty! Dare and try this for breakfast tomorrow!

Preparation time: 10 minutes
Cooking time: 10 minutes
Servings: 1

Ingredients:

- 4 ounces sirloin
- 1 small avocado, pitted, peeled and sliced
- 3 eggs
- 1 tablespoon ghee
- Salt and black pepper to the taste

Directions:

Heat up a pan with the ghee over medium high heat, crack eggs into the pan and cook them as you wish. Season with salt and pepper, take off heat and transfer to a plate. Heat up another pan over medium high heat, add sirloin, cook for 4 minutes, take off heat, leave aside to cool down and cut into thin strips. Season with salt and pepper to the taste and place next to the eggs. Add avocado slices on the side and serve.

Nutrition: calories 500, fat 34, fiber 10, carbs 3, protein 40

Amazing Chicken Omelet

It tastes amazing and it looks incredible! It's perfect!

Preparation time: 10 minutes
Cooking time: 10 minutes
Servings: 1

Ingredients:

- 1 ounce rotisserie chicken, shredded
- 1 teaspoon mustard
- 1 tablespoon homemade mayonnaise
- 1 tomato, chopped
- 2 bacon slices, cooked and crumbled
- 2 eggs
- 1 small avocado, pitted, peeled and chopped
- Salt and black pepper to the taste

Directions:

In a bowl, mix eggs with some salt and pepper and whisk gently. Heat up a pan over medium heat, spray with some cooking oil, add eggs and cook your omelet for 5 minutes. Add chicken, avocado, tomato, bacon, mayo and mustard on one half of the omelet. Fold omelet, cover pan and cook for 5 minutes more. Transfer to a plate and serve.

Nutrition: calories 400, fat 32, fiber 6, carbs 4, protein 25

Simple Smoothie Bowl

It's one of the best keto breakfast ideas ever!

Preparation time: 5 minutes
Cooking time: 0 minutes
Servings: 1

Ingredients:

- 2 ice cubes
- 1 tablespoon coconut oil
- 2 tablespoons heavy cream
- 1 cup spinach
- ½ cup almond milk
- 1 teaspoon protein powder
- 4 raspberries
- 1 tablespoon coconut ,shredded
- 4 walnuts
- 1 teaspoon chia seeds

Directions:

In your blender, mix milk with spinach, cream, ice, protein powder and coconut oil, blend well and transfer to a bowl. Top your bowl with raspberries, coconut, walnuts and chia seeds and serve.

Nutrition: calories 450, fat 34, fiber 4, carbs 4, protein 35

Feta Omelet

The combination of ingredients is just wonderful!

Preparation time: 10 minutes
Cooking time: 10 minutes
Servings: 1

Ingredients:
- 3 eggs
- 1 tablespoon ghee
- 1 ounce feta cheese, crumbled
- 1 tablespoon heavy cream
- 1 tablespoon jarred pesto
- Salt and black pepper to the taste

Directions:

In a bowl, mix eggs with heavy cream, salt and pepper and whisk well. Heat up a pan with the ghee over medium high heat, add whisked eggs, spread into the pan and cook your omelet until it's fluffy. Sprinkle cheese and spread pesto on your omelet, fold in half, cover pan and cook for 5 minutes more. Transfer omelet to a plate and serve.

Nutrition: calories 500, fat 43, fiber 6, carbs 3, protein 30

Breakfast Meatloaf

This is something worth trying as soon as possible!

Preparation time: 10 minutes
Cooking time: 35 minutes
Servings: 4

Ingredients:
- 1 teaspoon ghee
- 1 small yellow onion, chopped
- 1 pound sweet sausage, chopped
- 6 eggs
- 1 cup cheddar cheese, shredded
- 4 ounces cream cheese, soft
- Salt and black pepper to the taste
- 2 tablespoons scallions, chopped

Directions:

In a bowl, mix eggs with salt, pepper, onion, sausage and half of the cream and whisk well. Grease a meatloaf with the ghee, pour sausage and eggs mix, introduce in the oven at 350 degrees F and bake for 30 minutes. Take meatloaf out of the oven, leave aside for a couple of minutes, spread the rest of the cream cheese on top and sprinkle scallions and cheddar cheese all over. Introduce meatloaf in the oven again and bake for 5 minutes more. After the time has passed, broil meatloaf for 3 minutes, leave it aside to cool down a bit, slice and serve it.

Nutrition: calories 560, fat 32, fiber 1, carbs 6, protein 45

Breakfast Tuna Salad
You will love this Ketogenic breakfast from now on!

Preparation time: 10 minutes
Cooking time: 0 minutes
Servings: 4

Ingredients:
- 2 tablespoons sour cream
- 12 ounces tuna in olive oil
- 4 leeks, finely chopped
- Salt and black pepper to the taste
- A pinch of chili flakes
- 1 tablespoon capers
- 8 tablespoons homemade mayonnaise

Directions:
In a salad bowl, mix tuna with capers, salt, pepper, leeks, chili flakes, sour cream and mayo. Stir well and serve with some crispy bread.

Nutrition: calories 160, fat 2, fiber 1, carbs 2, protein 6

Incredible Breakfast Salad In A Jar
You can even take this at the office!

Preparation time: 10 minutes
Cooking time: 0 minutes
Servings: 1

Ingredients:
- 1 ounce favorite greens
- 1 ounce red bell pepper, chopped
- 1 ounce cherry tomatoes, halved
- 4 ounces rotisserie chicken, roughly chopped
- 4 tablespoons extra virgin olive oil
- ½ scallion, chopped
- 1 ounce cucumber, chopped
- Salt and black pepper to the taste

Directions:
In a bowl, mix greens with bell pepper, tomatoes, scallion, cucumber, salt, pepper and olive oil and toss to coat well. Transfer this to a jar, top with chicken pieces and serve for breakfast.

Nutrition: calories 180, fat 12, fiber 4, carbs 5, protein 17

Delicious Naan Bread And Butter

Try this special keto breakfast! It's so easy to make!

Preparation time: 10 minutes
Cooking time: 10 minutes
Servings: 6

Ingredients:

- 7 tablespoons coconut oil
- ¾ cup coconut flour
- 2 tablespoons psyllium powder
- ½ teaspoon baking powder
- Salt to the taste
- 2 cups hot water
- Some coconut oil for frying
- 2 garlic cloves, minced
- 3.5 ounces ghee

Directions:

In a bowl, mix coconut flour with baking powder, salt and psyllium powder and stir. Add 7 tablespoons coconut oil and the hot water and start kneading your dough Leave aside for 5 minutes, divide into 6 balls and flatten them on a working surface. Heat up a pan with some coconut oil over medium high heat, add naan breads to the pan, fry them until they are golden and transfer them to a plate. Heat up a pan with the ghee over medium high heat, add garlic, salt and pepper, stir and cook for 2 minutes. Brush naan breads with this mix and pour the rest into a bowl. Serve in the morning.

Nutrition: calories 140, fat 9, fiber 2, carbs 3, protein 4

Ketogenic Recipes For Lunch

Turkey Salad

This is packed with healthy elements and it's 100% keto!

Preparation time: 5 minutes
Cooking time: 0 minutes
Servings: 4

Ingredients:

- 1 cup cherry tomatoes, halved
- 1 cucumber, sliced
- 1 carrot, grated
- Salt and black pepper to the taste
- 1 tablespoon balsamic vinegar
- 1 tablespoon olive oil
- 1 and ½ cups turkey breast, cooked, skinless, boneless and shredded

Directions:

In a salad bowl, combine the turkey with the tomatoes, cucumber and the other ingredients, toss and serve for lunch.

Nutrition: calories 57, fat 3.7, fiber 1.3, carbs 6.1, protein 1.2

Cheesy Turkey Pan

It's an easy and tasty lunch idea for all those who are on a Keto diet!

Preparation time: 10 minutes
Cooking time: 25 minutes
Servings: 4

Ingredients:

- 2 cups cheddar cheese, grated
- 1 big turkey breast, skinless, boneless and cubed
- 1 tablespoon tomato passata
- ¼ cup veggie stock
- 1 tablespoon olive oil
- 2 shallots, chopped
- ¼ cup tomatoes, cubed
- Salt and black pepper to the taste

Directions:

Heat up a pan with the oil over medium heat, add the shallots and sauté for 2 minutes. Add the meat and brown for 5 minutes. Ad the passata and the other ingredients except the cheese, toss and cook over medium heat for 10 minutes more. Sprinkle the cheese on top, cook everything for 7-8 minutes, divide between plates and serve for lunch.

Nutrition: calories 309, fat 23.1, fiber 0.4, carbs 3.9, protein 21.6

Chicken and Leeks Pan

We recommend you to try this Ketogenic pizza for lunch today!

Preparation time: 10 minutes
Cooking time: 20 minutes
Servings: 4

Ingredients:

2 tablespoons olive oil
1 pound chicken breast, skinless, boneless and cut into strips
2 shallots, chopped
1 cup mozzarella cheese, shredded
2 leeks, sliced
½ cup veggie stock
1 tablespoon heavy cream
1 teaspoon sweet paprika
Salt and black pepper to the taste

Directions:

Heat up a pan with the oil over medium heat, add the shallots, stir and cook for 3 minutes. Add the meat and the leeks, stir and brown for 7 minutes more. Add the other ingredients except the cheese and stir. Sprinkle the cheese on top, introduce the pan in the oven and cook everything at 400 degrees F for 10 minutes more. Divide the mix between plates and serve.

Nutrition: calories 253, fat 12.9, fiber 1, carbs 7.2, protein 26.9

Chicken and Peppers Mix

This tastes so divine! They are so amazing!

Preparation time: 10 minutes
Cooking time: 25 minutes
Servings: 4

Ingredients:

- 1 cup red bell peppers, cut into strips
- 1 pound chicken breast, skinless, boneless and roughly cubed
- 2 spring onions, chopped
- 2 tablespoons olive oil
- 1 tomato, cubed
- Salt and black pepper to the taste
- ¼ cup tomato passata
- 1 tablespoon cilantro, chopped

Directions:

Heat up a pan with the oil over medium heat, add the spring onions and sauté them for 2 minutes   Add the chicken and the bell peppers, stir and cook everything for 8 minutes more. Add the rest of the ingredients, bring to a simmer and cook over medium heat for 15 minutes more stirring often. Divide the mix between plates and serve

Nutrition: calories 206, fat 10, fiber 0.9, carbs 3.7, protein 24.8

Paprika Chicken Mix

Get all the ingredients you need and make this amazing keto lunch as soon as possible!

Preparation time: 10 minutes
Cooking time: 25 minutes
Servings: 4

Ingredients:

- 1 cup mozzarella, shredded
- 2 tablespoons olive oil
- 2 shallots, chopped
- 1 pound chicken breast, skinless, boneless and roughly cubed
- 1 cup carrots, sliced
- 1 teaspoon sweet paprika
- ¼ teaspoon onion powder
- ¼ teaspoon garlic powder
- ½ cup chicken stock
- 1 tablespoon chives, chopped

Directions:

Heat up a pan with the oil over medium heat, add the shallots and sauté for 2 minutes. Add the carrots, paprika, onion and garlic powder, stir and sauté for 3 minutes more. Add the meat and brown it for 5 minutes more. Add the stock, sprinkle the cheese, cook everything for 15 minutes more. Sprinkle the chives on top, divide the mix between plates and serve.

Nutrition: calories 200, fat 4.5, fiber 3.5, carbs 8.5, protein 10

Beef Salad

It's so delicious! Why don't you try it today?

Preparation time: 10 minutes
Cooking time: 25 minutes
Servings: 4

Ingredients:

- 1 tablespoon lime juice
- 2 spring onions, chopped
- 2 shallots, chopped
- 2 garlic cloves, minced
- 2 tablespoons avocado oil
- 1 pound beef meat, ground
- 1 avocado, peeled, pitted and cubed
- 1 cup cherry tomatoes, halved
- 1 cup baby spinach
- A pinch of salt and black pepper
- ½ teaspoon hot paprika
- ¼ teaspoon chili powder
- 1 tablespoon cilantro, chopped
- 1 tablespoon chives, chopped

Directions:

Heat up a pan with the oil over medium heat, add the shallots, garlic and spring onions, stir and sauté for 5 minutes. Add the meat and brown for 5 minutes more. Add the rest of the ingredients, toss gently, cook everything over medium heat for 10 minutes more, divide into bowls and serve for lunch.

Nutrition: calories 340, fat 30, fiber 5, carbs 3, protein 32

Green Beans Salad
This is perfect for a Ketogenic lunch!

Preparation time: 10 minutes
Cooking time: 15 minutes
Servings: 4

Ingredients:

- 1 pound green beans, trimmed and halved
- 1 tablespoon olive oil
- 2 garlic cloves, minced
- 2 spring onions, chopped
- ½ cup tomato passata
- A pinch of salt and black pepper
- 1 cup cherry tomatoes, halved
- 1 cup baby spinach
- 1 tablespoon lime juice
- 1 tablespoon balsamic vinegar
- ½ teaspoon cumin, ground

Directions:

Heat up a pan with the oil over medium heat, add the garlic and the spring onions, stir and sauté for 2 minutes. Add the green beans and the other ingredients, bring everything to a simmer, cook over medium heat for 12 minutes, divide into bowls and serve for lunch.

Nutrition: calories 320, fat 8, fiber 4, carbs 3, protein 10

Beef Meatballs
These meatballs are really something very special!

Preparation time: 10 minutes
Cooking time: 14 minutes
Servings: 6

Ingredients:

- 2 pounds beef, ground
- 2 eggs, whisked
- 1 tablespoon garlic, minced
- 1 tablespoon sweet paprika
- 1 tablespoon cilantro, chopped
- 2 tablespoons almond meal
- 2 shallots, chopped
- 2 tablespoons olive oil

Directions:

In a bowl, mix the beef with the garlic, paprika and the other ingredients except the oil, stir and shape medium meatballs out of this mix. Heat up a pan with the oil over medium heat, add the meatballs, cook them for 6-7 minutes on each side, divide them between plates and serve for lunch.

Nutrition: calories 180, fat 8, fiber 1, carbs 4, protein 20

Chicken Meatballs and Sauce

We recommend you try this mix soon!

Preparation time: 10 minutes
Cooking time: 30 minutes
Servings: 4

Ingredients:

For the sauce:
- 2 shallots, chopped
- 1 tablespoon olive oil
- 1 cup tomato passata
- 4 garlic cloves, minced
- 1 tablespoon balsamic vinegar

For the meatballs:
- 2 pounds chicken meat, skinless, boneless and ground
- 2 eggs, whisked
- 2 spring onions, chopped
- 2 tablespoons almond flour
- 2 tablespoons cilantro, chopped

Directions:

In a bowl, combine the meat with the eggs, spring onions, flour and the cilantro, stir well and shape medium meatballs out of this mix. Heat up a pan with the oil over medium heat, add the meatballs, brown them for 2 minutes on each side and transfer them to a plate. Heat up the pan again over medium heat, add the shallots and the garlic, stir and cook for 5 minutes. Add the passata and the vinegar, stir and simmer the sauce for 3 minutes more. Add the meatballs, cook everything for 15 minutes more, divide into bowls and serve for lunch.

Nutrition: calories 340, fat 12.6, fiber 6.4, carbs 7, protein 12.5

Shrimp and Zucchini Pan

It's easy to make and very light! Try this lunch dish soon!

Preparation time: 5 minutes
Cooking time: 8 minutes
Servings: 4

Ingredients:
- 1 tablespoon olive oil
- 1 pound shrimp, peeled and deveined
- 1 cup zucchinis, sliced
- 2 shallots, chopped
- 1 tablespoon garlic, minced
- 1 tablespoon red chili flakes
- A pinch of salt and black pepper
- 1 tablespoon basil, chopped

Directions:

Heat up a pan with the oil and ghee over medium heat, add the shallots and the garlic, stir and sauté for 2 minutes. Add the shrimp, zucchinis and the other ingredients, cook everything for 6 minutes more, divide between plates and serve for lunch.

Nutrition: calories 176, fat 5.5, fiber 0.4, carbs 4.2, protein 26.5

Avocado and Zucchini Salad
It's so refreshing and healthy! We adore this salad!

Preparation time: 10 minutes
Cooking time: 0 minutes
Servings: 4

Ingredients:
- 1 cup arugula
- 1 avocado, peeled, pitted and cut into wedges
- 3 cups zucchini noodles
- ½ cup mozzarella, shredded
- 1 tablespoon avocado oil
- 1 tablespoon balsamic vinegar
- 1 cup cherry tomatoes, halved
- A pinch of salt and black pepper

Directions:
In a salad bowl, combine the zucchini noodles with the arugula and the other ingredients, toss and serve for lunch.

Nutrition: calories 141, fat 11.1, fiber 5.1, carbs 9.5, protein 3.6

Dill Salmon Salad
The best salmon salad you could taste is now available for you!

Preparation time: 10 minutes
Cooking time: 0 minutes
Servings: 2

Ingredients:
- ½ cup green onion, chopped
- 2 smoked salmon fillets, boneless, skinless and roughly shredded
- 2 tablespoons dill, chopped
- 1 avocado, peeled, pitted and roughly cubed
- ½ tablespoons balsamic vinegar
- 1 tablespoon olive oil
- Salt and black pepper to the taste
- 2 tablespoons prepared horseradish

Directions:
In a bowl, combine the salmon with the green onion and the other ingredients, toss and serve for lunch.

Nutrition: calories 467, fat 38.1, fiber 8.3, carbs 14.9, protein 4.3

Balsamic Steaks

If you are not in the mood for a Ketogenic steak, try this recipe!

Preparation time: 10 minutes
Cooking time: 15 minutes
Servings: 4

Ingredients:

- 1 pound beef steaks, cut into 4 sliced
- 2 tablespoons olive oil
- Salt and black pepper to the taste
- ¼ cup balsamic vinegar
- 2 garlic cloves, minced
- 1 teaspoon red pepper flakes
- 1 teaspoon garlic powder
- 2 shallots, chopped
- 1 tablespoon chives, chopped

Directions:

Heat up a pan with the oil over medium heat, add the garlic, shallots, pepper flakes and garlic powder, stir and sauté for 5 minutes. Add the steaks and the other ingredients, cook them for 5 minutes on each side, divide between plates and serve.

Nutrition: calories 435, fat 23, fiber 7, carbs 10, protein 35

Turkey and Endives Salad

Try each day a different lunch salad!

Preparation time: 10 minutes
Cooking time: 0 minutes
Servings: 4

Ingredients:

- 1 turkey breast, skinless, boneless, cooked and cut into strips
- 2 tablespoons avocado oil
- 2 endives, shredded
- 1 cup cherry tomatoes, halved
- 2 tablespoons lime juice
- 2 tablespoons balsamic vinegar
- 2 tablespoons chives, chopped
- Salt and black pepper to the taste

Directions:

In a bowl, mix the turkey with the endives and the other ingredients, toss and serve for lunch.

Nutrition: calories 200, fat 10, fiber 1.54, carbs 3, protein 7

Avocado Salad
It's so easy to make for lunch!

Preparation time: 5 minutes
Cooking time: 0 minutes
Servings: 2

Ingredients:

- 2 big avocados, pitted, peeled and cut into wedges
- 1 tablespoon olive oil
- 1 cup kalamata olives, pitted and halved
- 1 cup cucumber, sliced
- 1 tablespoon lime juice
- A pinch of salt and black pepper

Directions:

In a salad bowl, combine the avocados with the olives and the other ingredients, toss and serve cold for lunch.

Nutrition: calories 230, fat 13.4, fiber 12, carbs 5, protein 6.7

Chicken Stew
The combination is absolutely delicious! You should try it!

Preparation time: 10 minutes
Cooking time: 20 minutes
Servings: 4

Ingredients:

- 1 pound chicken breast, skinless, boneless and cubed
- 1 cup chicken stock
- ½ cup tomato passata
- 1 red onion, chopped
- 1 tablespoon avocado oil
- 1 red bell pepper, cubed
- 1 shallot, chopped
- A pinch of salt and black pepper
- 2 garlic cloves, minced
- 1 cup cherry tomatoes, halved
- 1 tablespoon cilantro, chopped

Directions:

Heat up a pan with the oil over medium heat, add the shallot and the garlic and sauté for 2 minutes. Add the meat and brown it for 3 minutes. Add the stock and the other ingredients, bring to a simmer and cook over medium heat for 15 minutes more, stirring from time to time. Divide the stew into bowls and serve for lunch.

Nutrition: calories 357, fat 23, fiber 5, carbs 6.3, protein 26

Beef and Radish Stew

It's delicious and you will adore it once you try it!

Preparation time: 10 minutes
Cooking time: 32 minutes
Servings: 4

Ingredients:

- 1 pound beef stew meat, cubed
- 2 shallots, chopped
- 2 tablespoons olive oil
- 2 garlic cloves, minced
- 1 cup radishes, cubed
- 1 cup black olives, pitted and halved
- 1 cup tomato passata
- 1 cup beef stock
- ½ teaspoon rosemary, dried
- ½ teaspoon oregano, dried
- 1 tablespoon parsley, chopped
- A pinch of salt and black pepper

Directions:

Heat up a pot with the oil over medium heat, add the shallot and the garlic and sauté for 2 minutes. Add the meat and brown for 5 minutes more. Add the radishes, olives and the other ingredients, bring to a simmer and cook over medium heat for 25 minutes more, stirring often. Divide the stew into bowls and serve.

Nutrition: calories 456, fat 32, fiber 2, carbs 6, protein 30

Salmon Bowls

You won't regret trying this!

Preparation time: 10 minutes
Cooking time: 15 minutes
Servings: 4

Ingredients:

- 1 pound salmon fillets, boneless, skinless and roughly cubed
- 1 cup chicken stock
- 2 spring onions, chopped
- 1 tablespoon olive oil
- 1 cup kalamata olives, pitted and halved
- 1 avocado, pitted, peeled and roughly cubed
- 1 cup baby spinach
- A pinch of salt and black pepper
- ¼ cup cilantro, chopped
- 1 tablespoon basil, chopped
- 1 teaspoon lime juice

Directions:

Heat up a pan with the oil over medium heat, add the spring onions and the salmon, toss gently and cook for 5 minutes. Add the olives and the other ingredients, and cook over medium heat for 10 minutes more. Divide the mix into bowls and serve for lunch.

Nutrition: calories 254, fat 17, fiber 1.9, carbs 6.1, protein 20

Beef and Kale pan

This will really get to your soul!

Preparation time: 10 minutes
Cooking time: 20 minutes
Servings: 4

Ingredients:

- 1 pound beef stew meat, cubed
- 1 red onion, chopped
- 1 tablespoon olive oil
- 2 garlic cloves, minced
- 1 cup kale, torn
- 1 cup beef stock
- 1 teaspoon chili powder
- ½ teaspoon sweet paprika
- 1 teaspoon rosemary, dried
- 1 tablespoon cilantro, chopped
- A pinch of salt and black pepper

Directions:

Heat up a pan with the oil over medium heat, add the onion and the garlic, stir and sauté for 2 minutes. Add the meat and brown it for 5 minutes. Add the rest of the ingredients, bring to a simmer and cook over medium heat for 13 minutes more. Divide the mix between plates and serve for lunch.

Nutrition: calories 160, fat 10, fiber 3, carbs 1, protein 12

Cheesy Pork Casserole

This is something you've been craving for a very long time

Preparation time: 10 minutes
Cooking time: 40 minutes
Servings: 4

Ingredients:

- 1 cup cheddar cheese, grated
- 2 eggs, whisked
- 1 pound pork loin, cubed
- 2 tablespoons avocado oil
- 2 shallots, chopped
- A pinch of salt and black pepper
- 3 garlic cloves, minced
- 1 cup red bell peppers, cut into strips
- ¼ cup heavy cream
- 1 tablespoon chives, chopped
- ½ teaspoon cumin, ground

Directions:

Heat up a pan with the oil over medium heat, add the shallots and the garlic and sauté for 2 minutes. Add the bell peppers and the meat, toss and cook for 5 minutes more. Add the cumin, salt, pepper, toss and take off the heat. In a bowl, mix the eggs with the cream and the cheese, whisk and pour over the pork mix. Sprinkle the chives on top, introduce the pan in the oven and cook at 380 degrees F for 30 minutes. Divide the mix between plates and serve for lunch.

Nutrition: calories 455, fat 34, fiber 3, carbs 3, protein 33

Thyme Chicken Mix

Enjoy something really easy for lunch!

Preparation time: 10 minutes
Cooking time: 20 minutes
Servings: 4

Ingredients:

- 1 pound chicken breast, skinless, boneless and cut into strips
- 1 tablespoon olive oil
- 2 spring onions, chopped
- 1 cup baby spinach
- 1 tablespoon thyme, chopped
- ½ cup tomato passata
- A pinch of salt and black pepper

Directions:

Heat up a pan with the oil over medium heat, add the spring onions and the meat and brown for 5 minutes. Add the rest of the ingredients, bring to a simmer and cook over medium heat for 15 minutes, stirring from time to time. Divide the mix into bowls and serve.

Nutrition: calories 380, fat 40, fiber 5, carbs 1, protein 17

Chicken Soup

You might end up adoring this soup! Try it at least once!

Preparation time: 10 minutes
Cooking time: 8 hours
Servings: 4

Ingredients:

- 1 pound chicken breast, skinless, boneless and cubed
- 2 tablespoons olive oil
- 2 shallots, chopped
- 2 zucchinis, sliced
- 1 quart chicken stock
- Juice from 1 lime
- 2 chili peppers chopped
- 2 tablespoons cilantro, chopped

Directions:

In a slow cooker, combine the meat with the oil, shallots and the other ingredients, put the lid on and cook on Low for 8 hours. Divide the soup into bowls and serve.

Nutrition: calories 300, fat 5, fiber 6, carbs 3, protein 26

Zucchini Soup

Try this Ketogenic soup really soon!

Preparation time: 10 minutes
Cooking time: 22 minutes
Servings: 4

Ingredients:

- 1 quart chicken stock
- 1 pound zucchinis, roughly cubed
- 1 tablespoon avocado oil
- 2 shallots, chopped
- ½ cup heavy cream
- 1 tablespoon dill, chopped
- A pinch of salt and black pepper
- 1 teaspoon ginger powder
- Juice of 1 lime

Directions:

Heat up a pot with the oil over medium heat, add the shallots, stir and sauté for 2 minutes. Add the zucchinis, stock, salt, pepper and the ginger powder, stir, bring to a simmer and cook for 15 minutes. Add the cream and lime juice, blend the soup using an immersion blender, heat it up over medium heat for 5 minutes more, divide into bowls, sprinkle the dill on top and serve for lunch.

Nutrition: calories 450, fat 34, fiber 4, carbs 8, protein 12

Lime Turkey Soup

This Ketogenic soup is simple and very tasty!

Preparation time: 10 minutes
Cooking time: 30 minutes
Servings: 4

Ingredients:

- 1 pound turkey breast, skinless, boneless and cubed
- 2 shallots, chopped
- 2 tablespoons olive oil
- 2 garlic cloves, minced
- 2 tomatoes, cubed
- 1 jalapeno pepper, chopped
- 6 cups chicken stock
- A pinch of salt and black pepper
- 1 red bell pepper, chopped
- 2 tablespoons parsley, chopped
- 1 tablespoon lime juice

Directions:

Heat up a pot with the oil over medium heat, add the shallots and the garlic and sauté for 2 minutes. Add the meat, tomatoes and the other ingredients except the parsley, bring to a simmer and cook over medium heat for 28 minutes. Ladle the soup into bowls, sprinkle the parsley on top and serve.

Nutrition: calories 287, fat 14, fiber 2, carbs 7, protein 25

Beef Curry

Have you ever tried a keto curry?

Preparation time: 10 minutes
Cooking time: 45 minutes
Servings: 4
Ingredients:

- 2 tablespoons olive oil
- 1 pound beef stew meat, cubed
- 2 shallots, chopped
- 1 cup beef stock
- 2 cups coconut milk
- 1 tablespoon lime juice
- 3 garlic cloves, minced
- 1 tablespoon cilantro, chopped
- 1 tablespoon ginger, grated
- 2 tablespoons red curry paste
- 1 teaspoon turmeric, ground
- 1 teaspoon cumin, ground

Directions:

Heat up a pot with the oil over medium high heat, add the shallots, garlic and the ginger, stir and sauté for 5 minutes. Add the meat and the curry paste, toss and brown for 5 minutes more. Add the stock and the other ingredients, bring to a simmer and cook over medium heat for 35 minutes, stirring often. Divide the curry into bowls and serve for lunch.

Nutrition: calories 430, fat 22, fiber 4, carbs 7, protein 53

Lunch Spinach Rolls

These will be ready in no time!

Preparation time: 20 minutes
Cooking time: 15 minutes
Servings: 16
Ingredients:

- 6 tablespoons coconut flour
- ½ cup almond flour
- 2 and ½ cups mozzarella cheese, shredded
- 2 eggs
- A pinch of salt
- 4 ounces cream cheese
- 6 ounces spinach, torn
- A drizzle of avocado oil
- A pinch of salt
- ¼ cup parmesan, grated
- Mayonnaise for serving

For the filling:

Directions:

Heat up a pan with the oil over medium heat, add spinach and cook for 2 minutes. Add parmesan, a pinch of salt and cream cheese, stir well, take off heat and leave aside for now. Put mozzarella cheese in a heat proof bowl and microwave for 30 seconds. Add eggs, salt, coconut and almond flour and stir everything. Place dough on a lined cutting board, place a parchment paper on top and flatten dough with a rolling pin. Divide dough into 16 rectangles, spread spinach mix on each and roll them into cigar shapes. Place all rolls on a lined baking sheet, introduce in the oven at 350 degrees F and bake for 15 minutes. Leave rolls to cool down for a few minutes before serving them with some mayo on top.

Nutrition: calories 500, fat 65, fiber 4, carbs 14, protein 32

Delicious Steak Bowl

It's an easy and fulfilling keto lunch! Try it!

Preparation time: 15 minutes
Cooking time: 8 minutes
Servings: 4
Ingredients:

- 16 ounces skirt steak
- 4 ounces pepper jack cheese, shredded
- 1 cup sour cream
- Salt and black pepper to the taste
- 1 handful cilantro, chopped
- A splash of chipotle adobo sauce

For the guacamole:

- ¼ cup red onion, chopped
- 2 avocados, pitted and peeled
- Juice from 1 lime
- 1 tablespoon olive oil
- 6 cherry tomatoes, chopped
- 1 garlic clove, minced
- 1 tablespoon cilantro, chopped

Directions:

Put avocados in a bowl and mash with a fork. Add tomatoes, red onion, garlic, salt and pepper and stir well. Add olive oil, lime juice and 1 tablespoon cilantro, stir again very well and leave aside for now. Heat up a pan over high heat, add steak, season with salt and pepper, cook for 4 minutes on each side, transfer to a cutting board, leave aside to cool down a bit and cut in thin strips. Divide steak into 4 bowls, add cheese, sour cream and guacamole on top and serve with a splash of chipotle adobo sauce.

Nutrition: calories 600, fat 50, fiber 6, carbs 5, protein 30

Meatballs And Pilaf

This is a Ketogenic lunch everyone can

Preparation time: 10 minutes
Cooking time: 30 minutes
Servings: 4
Ingredients:

- 12 ounces cauliflower florets
- Salt and black pepper to the taste
- 1 egg
- 1 pound lamb, ground
- 1 teaspoon fennel seed
- 1 teaspoon paprika
- 1 teaspoon garlic powder

- 1 small yellow onion, chopped
- 2 garlic cloves, minced
- 2 tablespoons coconut oil
- 1 bunch mint, chopped
- 1 tablespoon lemon zest
- 4 ounces goat cheese, crumbled

Directions:

Put cauliflower florets in your food processor, add salt and pulse well. Grease a pan with some of the coconut oil, heat up over medium heat, add cauliflower rice, cook for 8 minutes, season with salt and pepper to the taste, take off heat and keep warm. In a bowl, mix lamb with salt, pepper, egg, paprika, garlic powder and fennel seed and stir very well. Shape 12 meatballs and place them on a plate for now. Heat up a pan with the coconut oil over medium heat, add onion, stir and cook for 6 minutes. Add garlic, stir and cook for 1 minute. Add meatballs, cook them well on all sides and take off heat. Divide cauliflower rice on plates, add meatballs and onion mix on top, sprinkle mint, lemon zest and goat cheese at the end and serve.

Nutrition: calories 470, fat 43, fiber 5, carbs 4, protein 26

Delicious Broccoli Soup

Try this superb soup as soon as possible!

Preparation time: 10 minutes
Cooking time: 30 minutes
Servings: 4

Ingredients:
- 1 white onion, chopped
- 1 tablespoon ghee
- 2 cups veggie stock
- Salt and black pepper to the taste
- 2 cups water
- 2 garlic cloves, minced
- 1 cup heavy cream
- 8 ounces cheddar cheese, grated
- 12 ounces broccoli florets
- ½ teaspoon paprika

Directions:
Heat up a pot with the ghee over medium heat, add onion and garlic, stir and cook for 5 minutes. Add stock, cream, water, salt, pepper and paprika, stir and bring to a boil. Add broccoli, stir and simmer soup for 25 minutes. Transfer to your food processor and blend well. Add cheese and blend again. Divide into soup bowls and serve hot.

Nutrition: calories 350, fat 34, fiber 7, carbs 7, protein 11

Lunch Green Beans Salad

It will soon become one of your favorite keto salads!

Preparation time: 10 minutes
Cooking time: 5 minutes
Servings: 8

Ingredients:
- 2 tablespoons white wine vinegar
- 1 and ½ tablespoons mustard
- Salt and black pepper to the taste
- 2 pounds green beans
- 1/3 cup extra virgin olive oil
- 1 and ½ cups fennel, thinly sliced
- 4 ounces goat cheese, crumbled
- ¾ cup walnuts, toasted and chopped

Directions:
Put water in a pot, add some salt and bring to a boil over medium high heat. Add green beans, cook for 5 minutes and transfer them to a bowl filled with ice water. Drain green beans well and put them in a salad bowl. Add walnuts, fennel and goat cheese and toss gently. In a bowl, mix vinegar with mustard, salt, pepper and oil and whisk well. our this over salad, toss to coat well and serve for lunch.

Nutrition: calories 200, fat 14, fiber 4, carbs 5, protein 6

Pumpkin Soup

This keto soup is very creamy and textured! You should really try it for lunch today!

Preparation time: 10 minutes

Cooking time: 20 minutes

Servings: 6

Ingredients:

- ½ cup yellow onion, chopped
- 2 tablespoons olive oil
- 1 tablespoon chipotles in adobo sauce
- 1 garlic clove, minced
- 1 teaspoon cumin, ground
- 1 teaspoon coriander, ground
- A pinch of allspice
- 2 cups pumpkin puree
- Salt and black pepper to the taste
- 32 ounces chicken stock
- ½ cup heavy cream
- 2 teaspoons vinegar
- 2 teaspoons stevia

Directions:

Heat up a pot with the oil over medium heat, add onions and garlic, stir and cook for 4 minutes. Add stevia, cumin, coriander, chipotles and cumin, stir and cook for 2 minutes. Add stock and pumpkin puree, stir and cook for 5 minutes. Blend soup well using an immersion blender and then mix with salt, pepper, heavy cream and vinegar. Stir, cook for 5 minutes more and divide into bowls. Serve right away.

Nutrition: calories 140, fat 12, fiber 3, carbs 6, protein 2

Delicious Green Beans Casserole

This will impress you for sure!

Preparation time: 10 minutes

Cooking time: 35 minutes

Servings: 8

Ingredients:

- 1 pound green beans, halved
- Salt and black pepper to the taste
- ½ cup almond flour
- 2 tablespoons ghee
- 8 ounces mushrooms, chopped
- 4 ounces onion, chopped
- 2 shallots, chopped
- 3 garlic cloves, minced
- ½ cup chicken stock
- ½ cup heavy cream
- ¼ cup parmesan, grated
- Avocado oil for frying

Directions:

Put some water in a pot, add salt, bring to a boil over medium high heat, add green beans, cook for 5 minutes, transfer to a bowl filled with ice water, cool down, drain well and leave aside for now. In a bowl, mix shallots with onions, almond flour, salt and pepper and toss to coat. Heat up a pan with some avocado oil over medium high heat, add onions and shallots mix, fry until they are golden. Transfer to paper towels and drain grease. Heat up the same pan over medium heat, add ghee and melt it. Add garlic and mushrooms, stir and cook for 5 minutes. Add stock and heavy cream, stir, bring to a boil and simmer until it thickens. Add parmesan and green beans, toss to coat and take off heat. Transfer this mix to a baking dish, sprinkle crispy onions mix all over, introduce in the oven at 400 degrees F and bake for 15 minutes. Serve warm.

Nutrition: calories 155, fat, 11, fiber 6, carbs 8, protein 5

Simple Lunch Apple Salad

This is not just Ketogenic! It's also very tasty!

Preparation time: 10 minutes
Cooking time: 0 minutes
Servings: 4
Ingredients:

- 2 cups broccoli florets, roughly chopped
- 2 ounces pecans, chopped
- 1 apple, cored and grated
- 1 green onion stalk
- Salt and black pepper to the taste
- 2 teaspoons poppy seeds
- 1 teaspoon apple cider vinegar
- ¼ cup mayonnaise
- ½ teaspoon lemon juice
- ¼ cup sour cream

Directions:

In a salad bowl, mix apple with broccoli, green onion and pecans and stir. Add poppy seeds, salt and pepper and toss gently. In a bowl, mix mayo with sour cream, vinegar and lemon juice and whisk well. Pour this over salad, toss to coat well and serve cold for lunch!

Nutrition: calories 250, fat 23, fiber 4, carbs 4, protein 5

Brussels Sprouts Gratin

It's a dense and rich keto lunch idea!

Preparation time: 10 minutes
Cooking time: 35 minutes
Servings: 4
Ingredients:

- 2 ounces onions, chopped
- 1 teaspoon garlic, minced
- 6 ounces Brussels sprouts, chopped
- 2 tablespoons ghee
- 1 tablespoon coconut aminos
- Salt and black pepper to the taste
- ½ teaspoon liquid smoke

For the sauce:

- 2.5 ounces cheddar cheese, grated
- 1 tablespoon ghee
- ½ cup heavy cream
- ¼ teaspoon turmeric
- ¼ teaspoon paprika
- A pinch of xanthan gum

For the pork crust:

- 3 tablespoons parmesan
- 0.5 ounces pork rinds
- ½ teaspoon sweet paprika

Directions:

Heat up a pan with 2 tablespoons ghee over high heat, add Brussels sprouts, salt and pepper, stir and cook for 3 minutes. Add garlic and onion, stir and cook for 3 minutes more. Add liquid smoke and coconut aminos, stir, take off heat and leave aside for now. Heat up another pan with 1 tablespoon ghee over medium heat, add heavy cream and stir. Add cheese, black pepper, turmeric, paprika and xanthan gum, stir and cook until it thickens again. Add Brussels sprouts mix, toss to coat and divide into ramekins. In your food processor, mix parmesan with pork rinds and ½ teaspoon paprika and pulse well. Divide these crumbs on top of Brussels sprouts mix, introduce ramekins in the oven at 375 degrees F and bake for 20 minutes. Serve right away.

Nutrition: calories 300, fat 20, fiber 6, carbs 5, protein 10

Simple Asparagus Lunch

You only need a few ingredients and a few minutes of your time to make this simple and very tasty keto lunch!

Preparation time: 10 minutes
Cooking time: 10 minutes
Servings: 4

Ingredients:

- 2 egg yolks
- Salt and black pepper to the taste
- ¼ cup ghee
- 1 tablespoon lemon juice
- A pinch of cayenne pepper
- 40 asparagus spears

Directions:

In a bowl, whisk egg yolks very well. Transfer this to a small pan over low heat. Add lemon juice and whisk well. Add ghee and whisk until it melts. Add salt, pepper and cayenne pepper and whisk again well. Meanwhile, heat up a pan over medium high heat, add asparagus spears and fry them for 5 minutes. Divide asparagus on plates, drizzle the sauce you've made on top and serve.

Nutrition: calories 150, fat 13, fiber 6, carbs 2, protein 3

Simple Shrimp Pasta

This is so yummy!

Preparation time: 10 minutes
Cooking time: 10 minutes
Servings: 4

Ingredients:

- 12 ounces angel hair noodles
- 2 tablespoons olive oil
- Salt and black pepper to the taste
- 2 tablespoons ghee
- 4 garlic cloves, minced
- 1 pound shrimp, raw, peeled and deveined
- Juice from ½ lemon
- ½ teaspoon paprika
- A handful basil, chopped

Directions:

Put water in a pot, add some salt, bring to a boil, add noodles, cook for 2 minutes, drain them and transfer to a heated pan. Toast noodles for a few seconds, take off heat and leave them aside. Heat up a pan with the ghee and olive oil over medium heat, add garlic, stir and brown for 1 minute. Add shrimp and lemon juice and cook for 3 minutes on each side. Add noodles, salt, pepper and paprika, stir, divide into bowls and serve with chopped basil on top.

Nutrition: calories 300, fat 20, fiber 6, carbs 3, protein 30

Incredible Mexican Casserole

Try this Mexican Ketogenic lunch will surprise you for sure!

Preparation time: 10 minutes
Cooking time: 35 minutes
Servings: 6
Ingredients:

- 2 chipotle peppers, chopped
- 2 jalapenos, chopped
- 1 tablespoon olive oil
- ¼ cup heavy cream
- 1 small white onion, chopped
- Salt and black pepper to the taste
- 1 pound chicken thighs, skinless, boneless and chopped
- 1 cup red enchilada sauce
- 4 ounces cream cheese
- Cooking spray
- 1 cup pepper jack cheese, shredded
- 2 tablespoons cilantro, chopped
- 2 tortillas

Directions:

Heat up a pan with the oil over medium heat, add chipotle and jalapeno peppers, stir and cook for a few seconds. Add onion, stir and cook for 5 minutes. Add cream cheese and heavy cream and stir until cheese melts. Add chicken, salt, pepper and enchilada sauce, stir well and take off heat. Grease a baking dish with cooking spray, place tortillas on the bottom, spread chicken mix all over and sprinkle shredded cheese. Cover with tin foil, introduce in the oven at 350 degrees F and bake for 15 minutes. Remove the tin foil and bake for 15 minutes more. Sprinkle cilantro on top and serve.

Nutrition: calories 240, fat 12, fiber 5, carbs 5, protein 20

Delicious Asian Lunch Salad

Try this exotic lunch salad tomorrow!

Preparation time: 10 minutes
Cooking time: 15 minutes
Servings: 4
Ingredients:

- 1 pound beef, ground
- 1 tablespoon sriracha
- 2 tablespoons coconut aminos
- 2 garlic cloves, minced
- 10 ounces cole slaw mix
- 2 tablespoon sesame seed oil
- Salt and black pepper to the taste
- 1 teaspoon apple cider vinegar
- 1 teaspoon sesame seeds
- 1 green onion stalk, chopped

Directions:

Heat up a pan with the oil over medium heat, add garlic and brown for 1 minute. Add beef, stir and cook for 10 minutes. Add cole slaw mix, toss to coat and cook for 1minute. Add vinegar, sriracha, coconut aminos, salt and pepper, stir and cook for 4 minutes more. Add green onions and sesame seeds, toss to coat, divide into bowls and serve for lunch.

Nutrition: calories 350, fat 23, fiber 6, carbs 3, protein 20

Simple Buffalo Wings

You must try these for lunch if you are on a keto diet!

Preparation time: 10 minutes
Cooking time: 20 minutes
Servings: 2

Ingredients:

- 2 tablespoons ghee
- 6 chicken wings, cut in halves
- Salt and black pepper to the taste
- A pinch of garlic powder
- ½ cup hot sauce
- A pinch of cayenne pepper
- ½ teaspoon sweet paprika

Directions:

In a bowl, mix chicken pieces with half of the hot sauce, salt and pepper and toss well to coat. Arrange chicken pieces on a lined baking dish, introduce in preheated broiler and broil 8 minutes. Flip chicken pieces and broil for 8 minutes more. Heat up a pan with the ghee over medium heat. Add the rest of the hot sauce, salt, pepper, cayenne and paprika, stir and cook for a couple of minutes. Transfer broiled chicken pieces to a bowl, add ghee and hot sauce mix over them and toss to coat well. Serve them right away!

Nutrition: calories 500, fat 45, fiber 12, carbs 1, protein 45

Amazing Bacon And Mushrooms Skewers

You only need about 20 minutes to make this simple and very tasty lunch!

Preparation time: 10 minutes
Cooking time: 20 minutes
Servings: 6

Ingredients:

- 1 pound mushroom caps
- 6 bacon strips
- Salt and black pepper to the taste
- ½ teaspoon sweet paprika
- Some sweet mesquite

Directions:

Season mushroom caps with salt, pepper and paprika. Spear a bacon strip on a skewer's ends. Spear a mushroom cap and fold over bacon. Repeat until you obtain a mushroom and bacon braid. Repeat with the rest of the mushrooms and bacon strip. Season with sweet mesquite, place all skewers on preheated kitchen grill over medium heat, cook for 10 minutes, flip and cook for 10 minutes more. Divide on plates and serve for lunch with a side salad!

Nutrition: calories 110, fat 7, fiber 4, carbs 2, protein 10

Simple Tomato Soup

You only need 5 minutes to get your keto lunch ready!

Preparation time: 10 minutes
Cooking time: 5 minutes
Servings: 4

Ingredients:

- 1 quart canned tomato soup
- 4 tablespoons ghee
- ¼ cup olive oil
- ¼ cup red hot sauce
- 2 tablespoons apple cider vinegar
- Salt and black pepper to the taste
- 1 teaspoon oregano, dried
- 2 teaspoon turmeric, ground
- 8 bacon strips, cooked and crumbled
- A handful green onions, chopped
- A handful basil leaves, chopped

Directions:

Put tomato soup in a pot and heat up over medium heat. Add olive oil, ghee, hot sauce, vinegar, salt, pepper, turmeric and oregano, stir and simmer for 5 minutes. Take off heat, divide soup into bowls, top with bacon crumbles, basil and green onions.

Nutrition: calories 400, fat 34, fiber 7, carbs 10, protein 12

Bacon Wrapped Sausages

These are so delightful! You will really love this keto lunch!

Preparation time: 10 minutes
Cooking time: 30 minutes
Servings: 4

Ingredients:

- 8 bacon strips
- 8 sausages
- 16 pepper jack cheese slices
- Salt and black pepper to the taste
- A pinch of garlic powder
- ½ teaspoon sweet paprika
- 1 pinch of onion powder

Directions:

Heat up your kitchen grill over medium heat, add sausages, cook for a few minutes on each side, transfer to a plate and leave them aside for a few minutes to cool down. Cut a slit in the middle of each sausage to create pockets, stuff each with 2 cheese slices and season with salt, pepper, paprika, onion and garlic powder. Wrap each stuffed sausage in a bacon strip, secure with toothpicks, place on a lined baking sheet, introduce in the oven at 400 degrees F and bake for 15 minutes. Serve hot for lunch!

Nutrition: calories 500, fat 37, fiber 12, carbs 4, protein 40

Lunch Lobster Bisque

Are you looking for a special keto recipe to make for lunch? Try this next one!

Preparation time: 10 minutes
Cooking time: 1 hour
Servings: 4
Ingredients:

- 4 garlic cloves, minced
- 1 small red onion, chopped
- 24 ounces lobster chunks, pre-cooked
- Salt and black pepper to the taste
- ½ cup tomato paste
- 2 carrots, finely chopped
- 4 celery stalks, chopped
- 1 quart seafood stock
- 1 tablespoon olive oil
- 1 cup heavy cream
- 3 bay leaves
- 1 teaspoon thyme, dried
- 1 teaspoon peppercorns
- 1 teaspoon paprika
- 1 teaspoon xantham gum
- A handful parsley, chopped
- 1 tablespoon lemon juice

Directions:

Heat up a pot with the oil over medium heat, add onion, stir and cook for 4 minuets. Add garlic, stir and cook for 1 minute more. Add celery and carrot, stir and cook for 1 minute. Add tomato paste and stock and stir everything. Add bay leaves, salt, pepper, peppercorns, paprika, thyme and xantham gum, stir and simmer over medium heat for 1 hour. Discard bay leaves, add cream and bring to a simmer. Blend using an immersion blender, add lobster chunks and cook for a few minutes more. Add lemon juice, stir, divide into bowls and sprinkle parsley on top.

Nutrition: calories 200, fat 12, fiber 7, carbs 6, protein 12

Simple Halloumi Salad

Just gather all the ingredients you need and enjoy one of the best keto lunches!

Preparation time: 10 minutes
Cooking time: 10 minutes
Servings: 1
Ingredients:

- 3 ounces halloumi cheese, sliced
- 1 cucumber, sliced
- 1 ounce walnuts, chopped
- A drizzle of olive oil
- A handful baby arugula
- 5 cherry tomatoes, halved
- A splash of balsamic vinegar
- Salt and black pepper to the taste

Directions:

Heat up your kitchen grill over medium high heat, add halloumi pieces, grill them for 5 minutes on each side and transfer to a plate. In a bowl, mix tomatoes with cucumber, walnuts and arugula. Add halloumi pieces on top, season everything with salt, pepper, drizzle the oil and the vinegar, toss to coat and serve.

Nutrition: calories 450, fat 43, fiber 5, carbs 4, protein 21

Lunch Stew
It's so hearty and delicious! Trust us!

Preparation time: 10 minutes
Cooking time: 3 hours and 30 minutes
Servings: 6
Ingredients:

- 8 tomatoes, chopped
- 5 pounds beef shanks
- 3 carrots, chopped
- 8 garlic cloves, minced
- 2 onions, chopped
- 2 cups water
- 1 quart chicken stock
- ¼ cup tomato sauce
- 2 tablespoons apple cider vinegar
- 3 bay leaves
- 3 teaspoons red pepper, crushed
- 2 teaspoons parsley, dried
- 2 teaspoons basil, dried
- 2 teaspoons garlic powder
- 2 teaspoons onion powder
- A pinch of cayenne pepper

Directions:

Heat up a pot over medium heat, add garlic, carrots and onions, stir and brown for a few minutes. Heat up a pan over medium heat, add beef shank, brown for a few minutes on each side and take off heat. Add stock over carrots, the water and the vinegar and stir. Add tomatoes, tomato sauce, salt, pepper, cayenne pepper, crushed pepper, bay leaves, basil, parsley, onion powder and garlic powder and stir everything. Add beef shanks, cover pot, bring to a simmer and cook for 3 hours. Discard bay leaves, divide into bowls and serve.

Nutrition: calories 500, fat 22, fiber 4, carbs 6, protein 56

Chicken And Shrimp
It's a great combination! You'll see!

Preparation time: 10 minutes
Cooking time: 20 minutes
Servings: 2
Ingredients:

- 20 shrimp, raw, peeled
- 2 chicken breasts, boneless
- 2 handfuls spinach leaves
- ½ pound mushrooms, chopped
- Salt and black pepper to the taste
- ¼ cup mayonnaise
- 2 tablespoons sriracha
- 2 teaspoons lime juice
- 1 tablespoon coconut oil
- ½ teaspoon red pepper, crushed
- 1 teaspoon garlic powder
- ½ teaspoon paprika
- ¼ teaspoon xantham gum
- 1 green onion stalk, chopped

Directions:

Heat up a pan with the oil over medium high heat, add chicken breasts, season with salt, pepper, red pepper and garlic powder, cook for 8 minutes, flip and cook for 6 minutes more. Add mushrooms, more salt and pepper and cook for a few minutes. Heat up another pan over medium heat, add shrimp, sriracha, paprika, xantham and mayo, stir and cook until shrimp turn pink. Take off heat, add lime juice and stir everything. Divide spinach on plates, divide chicken and mushroom, top with shrimp mix, garnish with green onions and serve.

Nutrition: calories 500, fat 34, fiber 10, carbs 3, protein 40

Green Soup

This is just awesome!

Preparation time: 10 minutes
Cooking time: 13 minutes
Servings: 6

Ingredients:

- 1 cauliflower head, florets separated
- 1 white onion, finely chopped
- 1 bay leaf, crushed
- 2 garlic cloves, minced
- 5 ounces watercress
- 7 ounces spinach leaves
- 1 quart veggie stock
- 1 cup coconut milk
- Salt and black pepper to the taste
- ¼ cup ghee
- A handful parsley, for serving

Directions:

Heat up a pot with the ghee over medium high heat, add garlic and onion, stir and brown for 4 minutes. Add cauliflower and bay leaf, stir and cook for 5 minutes. Add watercress and spinach, stir and cook for 3 minutes. Add stock, salt and pepper, stir and bring to a boil. Add coconut milk, stir, take off heat and blend using an immersion blender. Divide into bowls and serve right away.

Nutrition: calories 230, fat 34, fiber 3, carbs 5, protein 7

Caprese Salad

This is very well know world wide but did you know that it can be served when you are on a Ketogenic diet?

Preparation time: 5 minutes
Cooking time: 0 minutes
Servings: 2

Ingredients:

- ½ pound mozzarella cheese, sliced
- 1 tomato, sliced
- Salt and black pepper to the taste
- 4 basil leaves, torn
- 1 tablespoon balsamic vinegar
- 1 tablespoon olive oil

Directions:

Alternate tomato and mozzarella slices on 2 plates. Sprinkle salt, pepper, drizzle vinegar and olive oil. Sprinkle basil leaves at the end and serve.

Nutrition: calories 150, fat 12, fiber 5, carbs 6, protein 9

Salmon Soup

This is so creamy!

Preparation time: 10 minutes
Cooking time: 25 minutes
Servings: 4

Ingredients:

- 4 leeks, trimmed and sliced
- Salt and black pepper to the taste
- 2 tablespoons avocado oil
- 2 garlic cloves, minced
- 6 cups chicken stock
- 1 pound salmon, cut in small pieces
- 2 teaspoons thyme, dried
- 1 and ¾ cups coconut milk

Directions:

Heat up a pot with the oil over medium heat, add leeks and garlic, stir and cook for 5 minutes. Add thyme, stock, salt and pepper, stir and simmer for 15 minutes. Add coconut milk and salmon, stir and bring to a simmer again. Divide into bowls and serve right away.

Nutrition: calories 270, fat 12, fiber 3, carbs 5, protein 32

Amazing Halibut Soup

If you are following a keto diet, then you should try this lunch idea for sure!

Preparation time: 10 minutes
Cooking time: 30 minutes
Servings: 4

Ingredients:

- 1 yellow onion, chopped
- 1 pound carrots, sliced
- 1 tablespoon coconut oil
- Salt and black pepper to the taste
- 2 tablespoons ginger, minced
- 1 cup water
- 1 pound halibut, cut in medium chunks
- 12 cups chicken stock

Directions:

Heat up a pot with the oil over medium heat, add onion, stir and cook for 6 minutes. Add ginger, carrots, water and stock, stir bring to a simmer, reduce temperature and cook for 20 minutes. Blend soup using an immersion blender, season with salt and pepper and add halibut pieces. Stir gently and simmer soup for 5 minutes more. Divide into bowls and serve.

Nutrition: calories 140, fat 6, fiber 1, carbs 4, protein 14

Ketogenic Side Dish Recipes

Cabbage Sauté
Serve this with a steak!

Preparation time: 10 minutes
Cooking time: 15 minutes
Servings: 4

Ingredients:
- 1 big green cabbage head, roughly shredded
- 2 shallots, chopped
- 1 tablespoon olive oil
- ½ cup veggie stock
- ½ cup tomato passata
- 1 tablespoon dill, chopped

Directions:
Heat up a pan with the oil over medium heat, add the shallots and sauté for 2 minutes. Add the cabbage, stir and cook for 3 minutes more. Add the rest of the ingredients, toss, bring to a simmer and cook over medium heat for 10 minutes more. Divide the sauté between plates and serve.

Nutrition: calories 97, fat 4, fiber 6, carbs 15.2, protein 3.5

Paprika Napa Cabbage
You will definitely enjoy this great side dish!

Preparation time: 10 minutes
Cooking time: 20 minutes
Servings: 4

Ingredients:
- 4 cups napa cabbage, roughly shredded
- 2 tablespoons avocado oil
- 2 spring onions, chopped
- ½ teaspoon garlic powder
- 1 teaspoon sweet paprika
- ½ cup veggie stock
- 1 tablespoon cilantro, chopped

Directions:
Heat up a pan with the oil over medium heat, add the spring onions, stir and sauté for 2 minutes. Add the cabbage and the other ingredients, toss, bring to a simmer and cook for 18 minutes more. Divide the mix between plates and serve.

Nutrition: calories 25, fat 1.4, fiber 1.5, carbs 3.3, protein 1.4

Cauliflower and Radish Mix

This simple Ketogenic sauté is awesome!

Preparation time: 10 minutes
Cooking time: 15 minutes
Servings: 4

Ingredients:

- ¼ cup veggie stock
- 1 tablespoon olive oil
- 3 garlic cloves, minced
- 1 cauliflower head, florets separated
- A pinch of salt and black pepper
- 1 cup radishes, cubed
- 2 tablespoons rosemary, chopped

Directions:

Heat up a pan with the oil over medium heat, add the garlic and sauté for 2 minutes. Add the cauliflower and the other ingredients, toss, bring to a simmer and cook over medium heat for 13 minutes more. Divide the mix between plates and serve as a side dish.

Nutrition: calories 61, fat 4, fiber 2.9, carbs 6.4, protein 1.7

Basil Zucchini and Tomatoes

These are simply the best! It's a great keto side dish!

Preparation time: 10 minutes
Cooking time: 18 minutes
Servings: 4

Ingredients:

- 2 zucchinis, roughly cubed
- ½ pound cherry tomatoes, halved
- 2 shallots, chopped
- 2 tablespoons olive oil
- ½ cup veggie stock
- A pinch of salt and black pepper
- 1 tablespoon basil, chopped
- 2 tablespoons balsamic vinegar

Directions:

Heat up a pan with the oil over medium heat, add the shallots, stir and sauté for 3 minutes. Add the zucchinis and the other ingredients, toss, cook over medium heat for 15 minutes more, divide between plates and serve.

Nutrition: calories 93, fat 7.5, fiber 1.8, carbs 6.7, protein 1.8

Sesame Green Beans

This is an amazing side dish you must try!

Preparation time: 10 minutes
Cooking time: 20 minutes
Servings: 4

Ingredients:

- 1 pound green beans, trimmed and halved
- 2 green onions, chopped
- 1 tablespoon avocado oil
- 2 garlic cloves, minced
- 1 tablespoon balsamic vinegar
- ½ cup chicken stock
- Salt and black pepper to the taste
- 1 teaspoon sesame seeds
- 1 tablespoon dill, chopped

Directions:

Heat up a pan with the oil over medium high heat, add the green onions and the garlic, stir and sauté for 2 minutes. Add the green beans and the other ingredients except the sesame seeds, toss, bring to a simmer and cook over medium heat for 18 minutes. Divide the mix between plates, sprinkle the sesame seeds on top and serve.

Nutrition: calories 110, fat 4, fiber 4, carbs 6, protein 4

Green Beans and Pine Nuts Mix

This can be served with a chicken dish!

Preparation time: 10 minutes
Cooking time: 15 minutes
Servings: 4

Ingredients:

- 2 tablespoons olive oil
- 1 pound green beans, trimmed and halved
- 2 tablespoons pine nuts
- 3 garlic cloves, minced
- ¼ cup parmesan cheese, grated
- 1 tablespoon cilantro, chopped
- A pinch of salt and black pepper

Directions:

Heat up a pan with the oil over medium heat, add the garlic and the pine nuts and cook for 5 minutes. Add the green beans, and the other ingredients, toss, cook for 10 minutes more, divide between plates and serve as a side dish.

Nutrition: calories 100, fat 7, fiber 3, carbs 5.1, protein 5

Balsamic Brussels Sprouts

You will love Brussels sprouts from now on!

Preparation time: 10 minutes
Cooking time: 20 minutes
Servings: 4

Ingredients:

- 1 pound Brussels sprouts, trimmed and halved
- 2 tablespoons olive oil
- A pinch of salt and black pepper
- ¼ teaspoon cumin, ground
- ½ teaspoon basil, dried
- 2 tablespoons balsamic vinegar
- 1 tablespoon cilantro, chopped

Directions:

In a roasting pan, combine the sprouts with the oil and the other ingredients, toss and bake at 400 degrees F for 20 minutes. Divide everything between plates and serve as a side dish.

Nutrition: calories 111, fat 7.4, fiber 4.3, carbs 10.5, protein 3.9

Cheesy Kale Sauté

This is very creamy and tasty!

Preparation time: 10 minutes
Cooking time: 20 minutes
Servings: 4

Ingredients:

- 2 shallots, chopped
- 2 garlic cloves, minced
- 1 pound kale, torn
- 1 tablespoon olive oil
- 1 cup heavy cream
- 1 tablespoon cilantro, chopped
- A pinch of salt and black pepper to the taste
- 2 tablespoons parmesan cheese, grated

Directions:

Heat up a pan with the oil over medium heat, add the shallots and the garlic, stir and sauté for 5 minutes. Add the kale and the other ingredients, toss, cook over medium heat for 15 minutes more, divide between plates and serve as a side dish.

Nutrition: calories 133, fat 10, fiber 4, carbs 4, protein 2

Cucumber Salad

Try this as a side dish for a delicious steak!

Preparation time: 10 minutes
Cooking time: 0 minutes
Servings: 4
Ingredients:

- 4 cucumbers, sliced
- 1 tablespoon olive oil
- 2 spring onions, chopped
- 1 tablespoon balsamic vinegar
- A pinch of cayenne pepper
- A pinch of salt and black pepper

Directions:

In a bowl, mix the cucumbers with the spring onions and the rest of the ingredients, toss and keep in the fridge for 10 minutes before serving as a side dish.

Nutrition: calories 150, fat 5.3, fiber 4, carbs 4.7, protein 7.6

Chili Cauliflower

This is so delicious and very easy to make at home! It's a great keto side dish!

Preparation time: 10 minutes
Cooking time: 30 minutes
Servings: 4
Ingredients:

- 1 pound cauliflower florets
- 1 teaspoon chili powder
- 2 tablespoons olive oil
- A pinch of salt and black pepper
- 1 tablespoon parsley, chopped

Directions:

In a roasting pan, combine the cauliflower with the other ingredients, toss and bake at 450 degrees F for 30 minutes. Divide the mix between plates and serve.

Nutrition: calories 118, fat 2, fiber 3, carbs 1, protein 6

Tomato and Peppers Salad

This is very simple and easy to make!

Preparation time: 10 minutes
Cooking time: 0 minutes
Servings: 4
Ingredients:

- 1 pound tomatoes, cut into wedges
- 2 red bell peppers, cut into strips
- 1 tablespoon lime juice
- 1 tablespoon olive oil
- 2 spring onions, chopped
- A pinch of salt and black pepper
- 1 tablespoon chives, chopped

Directions:

In a bowl, combine the peppers with the tomatoes and the other ingredients, toss and serve as a side dish.

Nutrition: calories 72, fat 3.9, fiber 2.4, carbs 9.5, protein 1.8

Parmesan Asparagus

This is a style keto side dish worth trying as soon as possible!

Preparation time: 10 minutes
Cooking time: 12 minutes
Servings: 4

Ingredients:

- 8 asparagus spears, trimmed and halved
- 2 tablespoons olive oil
- 2 garlic cloves, minced
- ½ cup veggie stock
- ½ teaspoons sweet paprika
- ¼ cup parmesan, grated
- 2 tablespoons lime juice

Directions:

Heat up a pan with the oil over medium high heat, add the garlic and sauté for 2 minutes. Add the asparagus, stock, paprika and lime juice, toss gently and cook over medium heat for 8 minutes more. Sprinkle the parmesan on top, cook the mix for 2 minutes more, divide between plates and serve.

Nutrition: calories 200, fat 4, fiber 6, carbs 2, protein 12

Minty Zucchinis

This side dish is not just a keto one! It's a simple and quick one as well!

Preparation time: 10 minutes
Cooking time: 15 minutes
Servings: 4

Ingredients:

- 1 pound zucchinis, sliced
- 1 tablespoon olive oil
- 2 garlic cloves, minced
- 1 tablespoon mint, chopped
- A pinch of salt and black pepper
- ¼ cup veggie stock

Directions:

Heat up a pan with the oil over medium high heat, add the garlic and sauté for 2 minutes. Add the zucchinis and the other ingredients, toss, cook everything for 10 minutes more, divide between plates and serve as a side dish.

Nutrition: calories 70, fat 1, fiber 1, carbs 0.4, protein 6

Chili Mustard Greens

This is just unbelievably amazing!

Preparation time: 10 minutes
Cooking time: 15 minutes
Servings: 4

Ingredients:

- 1 pound mustard greens
- 1 teaspoon chili powder
- 2 tablespoons olive oil
- 3 garlic cloves, minced
- ½ cup veggie stock
- A pinch of salt and black pepper
- 1 tablespoon red pepper flakes, crushed
- 1 tablespoon chives, chopped

Directions:

Heat up a pan with the oil over medium heat, add the garlic and sauté for 2 minutes. Add the mustard greens and the other ingredients, toss, bring to a simmer and cook over medium heat for 13 minutes more. Divide the mix between plates and serve as a side dish.

Nutrition: calories 143, fat 3, fiber 4, carbs 3, protein 4.6

Baked Tomato Mix

It's a keto side dish you will make over and over again!

Preparation time: 10 minutes
Cooking time: 25 minutes
Servings: 4

Ingredients:

- 1 pound tomatoes, cut into wedges
- 1 tablespoon balsamic vinegar
- 2 tablespoons olive oil
- A pinch of salt and black pepper
- 1 tablespoon basil, chopped

Directions:

Spread the tomatoes on a baking sheet lined with parchment paper, add the vinegar and the other ingredients, toss gently, and cook at 400 degrees F for 25 minutes. Divide between plates and serve hot as a side dish.

Nutrition: calories 55, fat 1, fiber 1, carbs 0.5, protein 7

Lime Brussels Sprouts
This side dish is perfect for a grilled steak!

Preparation time: 10 minutes
Cooking time: 25 minutes
Servings: 4
Ingredients:

- 1 pound Brussels sprouts, trimmed and halved
- 2 tablespoons lime juice
- 2 tablespoons avocado oil
- A pinch of salt and black pepper
- 1 teaspoon lime zest, grated
- 2 tablespoons basil, chopped

Directions:

In a roasting pan, combine the sprouts with the lime juice and the other ingredients, toss and bake at 400 degrees F for 25 minutes. Divide everything between plates and serve as a side dish.

Nutrition: calories 170, fat 15, fiber 4, carbs 4, protein 4

Celery Sauté
Serve this with some baked meat based dish!

Preparation time: 10 minutes
Cooking time: 20 minutes
Servings: 4
Ingredients:

- 2 tablespoons olive oil
- 3 celery stalks, roughly chopped
- 2 shallots, chopped
- ¼ cup veggie stock
- 1 tablespoon parmesan, grated
- A pinch of salt and black pepper

Directions:

Heat up a pan with the oil over medium-high heat, add the shallots and sauté for 3 minutes. Add the celery and the other ingredients, toss, cook everything over medium heat for 12 minutes more, divide between plates and serve.

Nutrition: calories 193, fat 14, fiber 3, carbs 6, protein 5

Grilled Asparagus
This Ketogenic side dish is perfect!

Preparation time: 10 minutes
Cooking time: 15 minutes
Servings: 4
Ingredients:

- 1 bunch asparagus spears, trimmed
- 2 tablespoons avocado oil
- 2 garlic cloves, minced
- 1 tablespoon lime juice
- A pinch of salt and black pepper

Direction:

In a bowl, combine the asparagus with the oil, garlic, salt and pepper and toss. Preheat the grill over medium heat, add the asparagus, cook for 6-7 minutes on each side, divide between plates, sprinkle the lime juice on top and serve.

Nutrition: calories 135, fat 11, fiber 4, carbs 6, protein 3

Kale and Brussels Sprouts Mix
Enjoy a great side dish!

Preparation time: 10 minutes
Cooking time: 15 minutes
Servings: 4

Ingredients:

- 1 pound Brussels sprouts, trimmed and halved
- 1 cup kale, torn
- 2 tablespoons olive oil
- 2 shallots, chopped
- ½ cup tomato passata
- A pinch of salt and black pepper
- 2 garlic cloves, minced
- 1 tablespoon cilantro, chopped

Directions:

Heat up a pan with the oil over medium heat, add the shallots and the garlic and sauté for 2 minutes. Add the sprouts and the other ingredients, bring to a simmer and cook over medium heat for 13 minutes more. Divide everything between plates and serve.

Nutrition: calories 70, fat 3, fiber 2, carbs 6, protein 4

Cumin Swiss Chard
You must try this keto side dish!

Preparation time: 10 minutes
Cooking time: 20 minutes
Servings: 4

Ingredients:

- 2 shallots, chopped
- 1 teaspoon cumin, ground
- 1 red bell pepper, cut into strips
- 1 bunch Swiss chard, roughly chopped
- 2 tablespoons lime juice
- 1 tablespoon olive oil
- A pinch of salt and black pepper

Directions:

Heat up a pan with the oil over medium heat, add the shallots and the bell pepper and sauté for 5 minutes. Add the Swiss chard and the other ingredients, bring to a simmer and cook over medium heat for 15 minutes more. Divide everything between plates and serve.

Nutrition: calories 300, fat 32, fiber 7, carbs 6, protein 8

Arugula Salad
This is really delicious and easy to make!

Preparation time: 10 minutes
Cooking time: 0 minutes
Servings: 4

Ingredients:
- 2 tablespoons olive oil
- 2 cups arugula
- 1 cup cherry tomatoes, halved
- ½ cup black olives, pitted and halved
- 1 avocado, peeled, pitted and cut into wedges
- 2 tablespoons lime juice
- A pinch of salt and black pepper

Directions:
In a bowl, combine the arugula with the tomatoes and the other ingredients, toss and serve as a side dish.

Nutrition: calories 160, fat 4, fiber 2, carbs 2, protein 6

Olives and Cucumber Salad
Get ready for a fabulous combination of ingredients!

Preparation time: 10 minutes
Cooking time: 0 minutes
Servings: 4

Ingredients:
- 1 cup black olives, pitted and halved
- 1 cup kalamata olives, pitted and halved
- 2 cucumbers, sliced
- 1 tablespoon olive oil
- 1 tablespoon balsamic vinegar
- 3 garlic cloves, minced
- 1 teaspoon basil, dried
- A pinch of salt and black pepper
- 1 tablespoons chives, chopped

Directions:
In a bowl, combine the olives with the cucumbers and the other ingredients, toss and serve as a side dish.

Nutrition: calories 200, fat 2, fiber 2, carbs 1, protein 10

Avocado Salsa
It's a simple keto side dish!

Preparation time: 10 minutes
Cooking time: 0 minutes
Servings: 4

Ingredients:
- 2 avocados, peeled, pitted and roughly cubed
- ¼ cup sun-dried tomatoes, drained and chopped
- 1 tablespoon lime juice
- 1 tablespoon avocado oil
- 2 red chilies, minced
- A pinch of salt and black pepper
- ¼ cup cilantro, finely chopped

Directions:
In a bowl, mix the avocados with the tomatoes and the other ingredients, toss and serve as a side dish.

Nutrition: calories 80, fat 1, fiber 2, carbs 1, protein 4

Cabbage and Avocado Salad
It's going to be the best side salad ever!

Preparation time: 10 minutes
Cooking time: 0 minutes
Servings: 4

Ingredients:
- 1 avocado, peeled, pitted and cubed
- 1 green cabbage head, shredded
- A pinch of salt and black pepper
- 2 tablespoons balsamic vinegar
- 2 tablespoons olive oil
- 1 garlic clove, minced
- 1 tablespoon cilantro, chopped

Directions:
In a bowl, combine the cabbage with the avocado and the other ingredients, toss and serve cold as a side dish.

Nutrition: calories 90, fat 0, fiber 2, carbs 2, protein 4

Cheesy Tomatoes and Zucchinis
This is rich and flavored!

Preparation time: 10 minutes
Cooking time: 20 minutes
Servings: 4

Ingredients:
- 1 pound cherry tomatoes, halved
- 3 zucchinis, sliced
- 2 tablespoons olive oil
- 1 tablespoon balsamic vinegar
- 2 garlic cloves, minced
- 1 tablespoon oregano, chopped
- A pinch of salt and black pepper
- ½ cup mozzarella, shredded

Directions:
In a roasting pan, combine the cherry tomatoes with the zucchinis and the other ingredients except the mozzarella and toss. Sprinkle the cheese on top, bake everything at 400 degrees F for 20 minutes, divide between plates and serve as a side dish.

Nutrition: calories 100, fat 2, fiber 2, carbs 1, protein 9

Fennel Salad
This is a very healthy keto side salad!

Preparation time: 10 minutes
Cooking time: 0 minutes
Servings: 4

Ingredients:
- 2 fennel bulbs, sliced
- 1 tablespoon lime juice
- 1 tablespoon olive oil
- ¼ cup walnuts, chopped
- 2 tablespoons chives, chopped
- A pinch of salt and black pepper

Directions:
In a bowl, combine the fennel with the lime juice and the other ingredients, toss and serve as a side salad.

Nutrition: calories 80, fat 0.2, fiber 1, carbs 0.4, protein 5

Spinach and Olives Salad

It's a good idea for a light keto side dish!

Preparation time: 10 minutes
Cooking time: 12 minutes
Servings: 4

Ingredients:

- ½ pound baby spinach
- 1 cup kalamata olives, pitted and halved
- 1 tablespoon olive oil
- 2 shallots, chopped
- 2 garlic cloves, minced
- ½ cup tomato passata
- 1 tablespoon cilantro, chopped
- A pinch of salt and black pepper

Directions:

Heat up a pan with the oil over medium heat, add the shallots and garlic, stir and sauté for 2 minutes. Add the spinach and the other ingredients, toss, cook over medium heat for 10 minutes more, divide between plates and serve.

Nutrition: calories 120, fat 3, fiber 2, carbs 1, protein 8

Herbed Tomatoes Mix

We really like this keto side dish!

Preparation time: 10 minutes
Cooking time: 30 minutes
Servings: 4

Ingredients:

- 1 pound mixed tomatoes, cut into wedges
- 2 tablespoons olive oil
- 1 tablespoon oregano, chopped
- 1 tablespoon basil, chopped
- 1 tablespoon chives, chopped
- 1 tablespoon rosemary, chopped
- 1 tablespoon balsamic vinegar
- A pinch of salt and black pepper

Directions:

In a roasting pan, combine tomatoes with the oil and the other ingredients, toss and bake at 380 degrees F for 30 minutes. Divide the tomatoes mix between plates and serve as a side dish.

Nutrition: calories 150, fat 1, fiber 2, carbs 1, protein 8

Special Endives And Watercress Side Salad

It's such a fresh side dish that goes with a keto grilled steak!

Preparation time: 10 minutes
Cooking time: 5 minutes
Servings: 4

Ingredients:

- 4 medium endives, roots and ends cut and thinly sliced crosswise
- 1 tablespoon lemon juice
- 1 shallot finely, chopped
- 1 tablespoon balsamic vinegar
- 2 tablespoons extra virgin olive oil
- 6 tablespoons heavy cream
- Salt and black pepper to the taste
- 4 ounces watercress, cut in medium springs
- 1 apple, thinly sliced
- 1 tablespoon chervil, chopped
- 1 tablespoon tarragon, chopped
- 1 tablespoon chives, chopped
- 1/3 cup almonds, chopped
- 1 tablespoon parsley, chopped

Directions:

In a bowl, mix lemon juice with vinegar, salt and shallot, stir and leave side for 10 minutes. Add olive oil, pepper, stir and leave aside for another 2 minutes. Put endives, apple, watercress, chives, tarragon, parsley and chervil in a salad bowl. Add salt and pepper to the taste and toss to coat. Add heavy cream and vinaigrette, stir gently and serve as a side dish with almonds on top.

Nutrition: calories 200, fat 3, fiber 5, carbs 2, protein 10

Indian Side Salad

It's very healthy and rich!

Preparation time: 15 minutes
Cooking time: 0 minutes
Servings: 6

Ingredients:

- 3 carrots, finely grated
- 2 courgettes, finely sliced
- A bunch of radishes, finely sliced
- ½ red onion, chopped
- 6 mint leaves, roughly chopped

For the salad dressing:

- 1 teaspoon mustard
- 1 tablespoons homemade mayo
- 1 tablespoons balsamic vinegar
- 2 tablespoons extra virgin olive oil
- Salt and black pepper to the taste

Directions:

In a bowl, mix mustard with mayo, vinegar, salt and pepper to the taste and stir well. Add oil gradually and whisk everything. In a salad bowl, mix carrots with radishes, courgettes and mint leaves. Add salad dressing, toss to coat and keep in the fridge until you serve it.

Nutrition: calories 140, fat 1, fiber 2, carbs 1, protein 7

Indian Mint Chutney

It has such a unique color and taste! It's a special side for any steak!

Preparation time: 10 minutes
Cooking time: 0 minutes
Servings: 8

Ingredients:

- 1 and ½ cup mint leaves
- 1 big bunch cilantro
- Salt and black pepper to the taste
- 1 green chili pepper, seedless
- 1 yellow onion, cut in medium chunks
- ¼ cup water
- 1 tablespoon tamarind juice

Directions:

Put mint and coriander leaves in your food processor and blend them. Add chili pepper, salt, black pepper, onion and tamarind paste and blend again. Add water, blend some more until you obtain a cream, transfer to a bowl and serve as a side for a tasty keto steak.

Nutrition: calories 100, fat 1, fiber 1, carbs 0.4, protein 6

Indian Coconut Chutney

It's perfect for a fancy Indian style Ketogenic dish!

Preparation time: 5 minutes
Cooking time: 5 minutes
Servings: 3

Ingredients:

- ½ teaspoon cumin
- ½ cup coconut, grated
- 2 tablespoons already fried chana dal
- 2 green chilies
- Salt to the taste
- 1 garlic clove
- ¾ tablespoons avocado oil
- ¼ teaspoon mustard seeds
- A pinch of hing
- ½ teaspoons urad dal
- 1 red chili chopped
- 1 spring curry leaves

Directions:

In your food processor, mix coconut with salt to the taste, cumin, garlic, chana dal and green chilies and blend well. Add a splash of water and blend again. Heat up a pan with the oil over medium heat, add red chili, urad dal, mustard seeds, hing and curry leaves, stir and cook for 2-3 minutes. Add this to coconut chutney, stir gently and serve as a side.

Nutrition: calories 90, fat 1, fiber 1, carbs 1, protein 6

Easy Tamarind Chutney

It's sweet and it's perfectly balanced! It's one of the best sides for a keto dish!

Preparation time: 10 minutes
Cooking time: 35 minutes
Servings: 10

Ingredients:

- 1 teaspoon cumin seeds
- 1 tablespoon canola oil
- ½ teaspoon garam masala
- ½ teaspoon asafetida powder
- 1 teaspoon ground ginger
- ½ teaspoon fennel seeds
- ½ teaspoon cayenne pepper
- 1 and ¼ cups coconut sugar
- 2 cups water
- 3 tablespoons tamarind paste

Directions:

Heat up a pan with the oil over medium heat, add ginger, cumin, cayenne pepper, asafetida powder, fennel seeds and garam masala, stir and cook for 2 minutes. Add water, sugar and tamarind paste, stir, bring to a boil, reduce heat to low and simmer chutney for 30 minutes. Transfer to a bowl and leave it to cool down before you serve it as a side for a steak.

Nutrition: calories 120, fat 1, fiber 3, carbs 5, protein 9

Caramelized Bell Peppers

A Ketogenic pork dish will taste much better with such a side dish!

Preparation time: 10 minutes
Cooking time: 32 minutes
Servings: 4

Ingredients:

- 1 tablespoon olive oil
- 1 teaspoon ghee
- 2 red bell peppers, cut in thin strips
- 2 red onions, cut in thin strips
- Salt and black pepper to the taste
- 1 teaspoon basil, dried

Directions:

Heat up a pan with the ghee and the oil over medium heat, add onion and bell peppers, stir and cook fro 2 minutes. Reduce temperature and cook for 30 minutes more stirring often. Add salt, pepper and basil, stir again, take off heat and serve as a keto side dish.

Nutrition: calories 97, fat 4, fiber 2, carbs 6, protein 2

Caramelized Red Chard

This is an easy side for a dinner dish!

Preparation time: 10 minutes
Cooking time: 20 minutes
Servings: 4
Ingredients:

- 2 tablespoons olive oil
- 1 yellow onion, chopped
- 2 tablespoons capers
- Juice from 1 lemon
- Salt and black pepper to the taste
- 1 teaspoon palm sugar
- 1 bunch red chard, chopped
- ¼ cup kalamata olives, pitted

Directions:

Heat up a pan with the oil over medium heat, add onions, stir and brown for 4 minutes. Add palm sugar and stir well. Add olives and chard, stir and cook for 10 minutes more. Add capes, lemon juice, salt and pepper, stir and cook for 3 minutes more. Divide on plates and serve as a keto side.

Nutrition: calories 119, fat 7, fiber 3, carbs 7, protein 2

Special Summer Kale Side Dish

This is perfect as a keto side dish for a summer delight!

Preparation time: 10 minutes
Cooking time: 45 minutes
Servings: 4
Ingredients:

- 2 cups water
- 1 tablespoon balsamic vinegar
- 1/3 cup almonds, toasted
- 3 garlic cloves, minced
- 1 bunch kale, steamed and chopped
- 1 small yellow onion, chopped
- 2 tablespoons olive oil

Directions:

Heat up a pan with the oil over medium heat, add onion, stir and cook for 10 minutes. Add garlic, stir and cook for 1 minute. Add water and kale, cover pan and cook for 30 minutes. Add salt, pepper, balsamic vinegar and almonds, toss to coat, divide on plates and serve as a side.

Nutrition: calories 170, fat 11, fiber 3, carbs 7, protein 7

Simple Fried Cabbage

The cabbage is such a versatile veggie! Try this amazing side dish as soon as possible!

Preparation time: 10 minutes
Cooking time: 15 minutes
Servings: 4
Ingredients:

- 1 and ½ pound green cabbage, shredded
- 3.5 ounces ghee

Directions:

Heat up a pan with the ghee over medium heat. Add cabbage and cook for 15 minutes stirring often. Add salt, pepper and paprika, stir, cook for 1 minute more, divide on plates and serve.

Nutrition: calories 200, fat 4, fiber 2, carbs 3, protein 7

Amazing Coleslaw

Coleslaws are very famous! Today, we recommend you a keto one!

Preparation time: 10 minutes
Cooking time: 0 minutes
Servings: 4

Ingredients:

- 1 small green cabbage head, shredded
- Salt and black pepper to the taste
- 6 tablespoons mayonnaise
- Salt and black pepper to the taste
- 1 pinch fennel seed
- Juice from ½ lemon
- 1 tablespoon Dijon mustard

Directions:

In a bowl, mix cabbage with salt and lemon juice, stir well and leave aside for 10 minutes. Press well the cabbage, add more salt and pepper, fennel seed, mayo and mustard. Toss to coat and serve.

Nutrition: calories 150, fat 3, fiber 2, carbs 2, protein 7

Delicious Green Beans And Avocado

Serve this with a tasty fish dish!

Preparation time: 10 minutes
Cooking time: 5 minutes
Servings: 4

Ingredients:

- 2/3 pound green beans, trimmed
- Salt and black pepper to the taste
- 3 tablespoons olive oil
- 2 avocados, pitted and peeled
- 5 scallions, chopped
- A handful cilantro, chopped

Directions:

Heat up a pan with the oil over medium heat, add green beans, stir and cook for 4 minutes. Add salt and pepper, stir, take off heat and transfer to a bowl. In another bowl, mix avocados with salt and pepper and mash with a fork. Add onions and stir well. Add this over green beans, toss to coat and serve with chopped cilantro on top.

Nutrition: calories 200, fat 5, fiber 3, carbs 4, protein 6

Creamy Spaghetti Pasta

This is just perfect for a turkey dish!

Preparation time: 10 minutes
Cooking time: 40 minutes
Servings: 4

Ingredients:

- 1 spaghetti squash
- Salt and black pepper to the taste
- 2 tablespoons ghee
- 1 teaspoon Cajun seasoning
- A pinch of cayenne pepper
- 2 cups heavy cream

Directions:

Prick spaghetti with a fork, place on a lined baking sheet, introduce in the oven at 350 degrees F and bake for 15 minutes. Take spaghetti squash out of the oven, leave aside to cool down a bit and scoop squash noodles. Heat up a pan with the ghee over medium heat, add spaghetti squash, stir and cook for a couple of minutes. Add salt, pepper, cayenne pepper and Cajun seasoning, stir and cook for 1 minute. Add heavy cream, stir, cook for 10 minutes more, divide on plates and serve as a keto side dish.

Nutrition: calories 200, fat 2, fiber 1, carbs 5, protein 8

Amazing Roasted Olives

This is a great side dish! You'll see!

Preparation time: 10 minutes
Cooking time: 20 minutes
Servings: 6

Ingredients:

- 1 cup black olives, pitted
- 1 cup kalamata olives, pitted
- 1 cup green olives, stuffed with almonds and garlic
- ¼ cup olive oil
- 10 garlic cloves
- 1 tablespoon herbes de Provence
- 1 teaspoon lemon zest, grated
- Black pepper to the taste
- Some chopped thyme for serving

Directions:

Place black, kalamata and green olives on a lined baking sheet, drizzle oil, garlic and herbes de Provence, toss to coat, introduce in the oven at 425 degrees F and bake for 10 minutes. Stir olives and bake for 10 minutes more. Divide olives on plates, sprinkle lemon zest, black pepper and thyme on top, toss to coat and serve warm.

Nutrition: calories 200, fat 20, fiber 4, carbs 3, protein 1

Delicious Veggie Noodles
These are very delicious and incredibly colored!

Preparation time: 10 minutes
Cooking time: 20 minutes
Servings: 6

Ingredients:
- 1 zucchini, cut with a spiralizer
- 1 summer squash, cut with a spiralizer
- 1 carrot, cut with a spiralizer
- 1 sweet potato, cut with a spiralizer
- 4 ounces red onion, chopped
- 6 ounces yellow, orange and red bell peppers, cut in thin strips
- Salt and black pepper to the taste
- 4 tablespoons bacon fat
- 3 garlic cloves, minced

Directions:
Spread zucchini noodles on a lined baking sheet. Add squash, carrot, sweet potato, onion and all bell peppers. Add salt, pepper and garlic and toss to coat. Add bacon fat, toss again all noodles, introduce in the oven at 400 degrees F and bake for 20 minutes. Transfer to plates and serve right away as a keto side dish.

Nutrition: calories 50, fat 1, fiber 1, carbs 6, protein 2

Mustard And Garlic Brussels Sprouts
We know a lot of great keto Brussels sprouts sides, but this is one of our favorite ones!

Preparation time: 10 minutes
Cooking time: 40 minutes
Servings: 4

Ingredients:
- 1 pound Brussels sprouts, trimmed and halved
- Salt and black pepper to the taste
- 1 tablespoon coconut aminos
- 1 tablespoon Dijon mustard
- 1 tablespoon garlic cloves, minced
- 1 tablespoons ghee
- 1 garlic clove head, cloves peeled and separated
- 1 tablespoon caraway seeds

Directions:
Put Brussels sprouts on a lined baking sheet. Add minced garlic, whole garlic, ghee, mustard, salt, pepper, coconut aminos and caraway seeds. Toss to coat very well, introduce in the oven at 400 degrees F and bake for 40 minutes. Transfer to plates and serve as a side for a roast.

Nutrition: calories 70, fat 4, fiber 2, carbs 4, protein 2.4

Amazing Cheese Sauce

It goes perfectly with meat and fish based dishes!

Preparation time: 10 minutes
Cooking time: 12 minutes
Servings: 8

Ingredients:

- 2 tablespoons ghee
- ¼ cup cream cheese, soft
- ¼ cup whipping cream
- ¼ cup cheddar cheese, grated
- 2 tablespoons water
- A pinch of salt
- ¼ teaspoon cayenne pepper
- ½ teaspoon sweet paprika
- ½ teaspoon onion powder
- ½ teaspoon garlic powder
- 4 tablespoons parsley, chopped

Directions:

Heat up a pan with the ghee over medium heat. Add whipping cream and stir well. Add cream cheese, stir and bring to a simmer. Take off heat, add cheddar cheese, stir, return to medium heat and cook for 3-4 minutes. Add the water, a pinch of sat, cayenne pepper, onion and garlic powder, paprika and parsley, stir well, take off heat and serve on top of meat or fished based meals.

Nutrition: calories 200, fat 13, fiber 0, carbs 1, protein 6

Kohlrabi Sauté

Have you ever heard of such a tasty keto side dish? Pay attention and learn how to make this simple dish!

Preparation time: 10 minutes
Cooking time: 10 minutes
Servings: 4

Ingredients:

- 2 kohlrabi, trimmed and thinly sliced
- Salt and black pepper to the taste
- 1 tablespoons parsley, chopped
- 1 tablespoon ghee
- 2 garlic cloves, minced

Directions:

Put some water in a pot and bring to a boil over medium heat. Add kohlrabi slices, cook for 5 minutes, drain and transfer to a bowl. Heat up a pan with the ghee over medium heat. Add garlic, stir and cook for 1 minute.Add kohlrabi slices, salt, pepper and cook until they are gold on both sides. Add parsley, toss to coat, transfer to plates and serve warm.

Nutrition: calories 87, fat 2.4, fiber 3, carbs 5, protein 4

Delicious Turnip Fries

You can make these fries really fast and they taste amazing!

Preparation time: 10 minutes
Cooking time: 25 minutes
Servings: 4

Ingredients:

- 2 pounds turnips, peeled and cut into sticks
- Salt to the taste
- ¼ cup olive oil

For the seasoning mix:

- 2 tablespoons chili powder
- 1 teaspoon garlic powder
- ½ teaspoon oregano, dried
- 1 and ½ teaspoons onion powder
- 1 and ½ tablespoons cumin, ground

Directions:

In a bowl, mix chili powder with onion and garlic one, cumin and oregano and stir well. Add parsnips sticks, rub them well and spread on a lined baking sheet. Season with salt, drizzle the oil, toss to coat well and bake in the oven at 350 degrees F for 25 minutes. Leave parsnip fries to cool down a bit before serving them as a keto side dish.

Nutrition: calories 140, fat 2, fiber 1, carbs 1, protein 6

Amazing Irish Side Dish

This is so amazing and fresh!

Preparation time: 10 minutes
Cooking time: 15 minutes
Servings: 6

Ingredients:

- 1 cup spinach leaves
- 3 cups cauliflower florets
- ¼ cup cream
- 4 tablespoons ghee
- Salt and black pepper to the taste
- ½ cup sour cream
- 1 avocado, pitted and peeled

Directions:

In a heat proof bowl, mix spinach with cauliflower florets, introduce in your microwave and cook for 15 minutes. Mash avocado with a fork and add to spinach mix. Also add salt, pepper, cream, ghee and sour cream and blend using an immersion blender. Transfer to plates and serve with a steak.

Nutrition: calories 190, fat 16, fiber 7, carbs 3, protein 5

Twice Baked Zucchinis
Serve this with a lamb dish and

Preparation time: 10 minutes
Cooking time: 30 minutes
Servings: 4

Ingredients:

- 2 zucchinis, cut in halves and each half in half lengthwise
- ¼ cup yellow onion, chopped
- ½ cup cheddar cheese, shredded
- 4 bacon strips, cooked and crumbled
- ¼ cup sour cream
- 2 ounces cream cheese, soft
- 1 tablespoon jalapeno pepper, chopped
- Salt and black pepper to the taste
- 2 tablespoons ghee

Directions:
Scoop zucchini insides, place flesh in a bowl and arrange zucchini cups in a baking dish. Add onion, cheddar cheese, bacon crumbles, jalapeno, salt, pepper, sour cream, cream cheese and ghee to the bowl. Whisk very well, fill zucchini quarters with this mix, introduce in the oven at 350 degrees F and bake for 30 minutes. Divide zucchinis on plates and serve with some lamb chops on the side.

Nutrition: calories 260, fat 22, fiber 4, carbs 3, protein 10

Delicious Gravy
This Ketogenic side sauce is out of this world!

Preparation time: 10 minutes
Cooking time: 10 minutes
Servings: 4

Ingredients:

- 4 ounces sausages, chopped
- Salt and black pepper to the taste
- 1 cup heavy cream
- 2 tablespoons ghee
- ½ teaspoon guar gum

Directions:
Heat up a pan over medium heat, add sausage pieces, stir, cook for 4 minutes and transfer to a plate. Return pan to medium heat, add ghee and melt it. Add cream, salt, pepper and guar gum, stir and cook until it begins to thicken. Return sausage to pan, stir well, take off heat and drizzle over a tasty keto steak.

Nutrition: calories 345, fat 34, fiber 0, carbs 2, protein 4

Mushroom And Hemp Pilaf

It's a very interesting and delicious side dish!

Preparation time: 10 minutes
Cooking time: 20 minutes
Servings: 4

Ingredients:

- 2 tablespoons ghee
- ¼ cup almonds, sliced
- 3 mushrooms, roughly chopped
- 1 cup hemp seeds
- Salt and black pepper to the taste
- ½ teaspoon garlic powder
- ½ cup chicken stock
- ¼ teaspoon parsley, dried

Directions:

Heat up a pan with the ghee over medium heat, add almonds and mushrooms, stir and cook for 4 minutes. Add hemp seeds and stir. Add salt, pepper, parsley, garlic powder and stock, stir, reduce heat, cover pan and simmer until stock is absorbed. Divide on plates and serve as a side dish.

Nutrition: calories 324, fat 24, fiber 15, carbs 2, protein 15

Asian Side Salad

It has a delicious and amazing flavor! It goes perfectly with some keto shrimp!

Preparation time: 30 minutes
Cooking time: 10 minutes
Servings: 4

Ingredients:

- 1 big cucumber, thinly sliced
- 1 spring onion, chopped
- 2 tablespoons coconut oil
- 1 packet Asian noodles
- 1 tablespoon balsamic vinegar
- 1 tablespoon sesame oil
- ¼ teaspoon red pepper flakes
- Salt and black pepper to the taste
- 1 teaspoon sesame seeds

Directions:

Cook noodles according to package instructions, drain and rinse them well. Heat up a pan with the coconut oil over medium high heat, add noodles, cover pan and fry them for 5 minutes until they are crispy enough. Transfer them to paper towels and drain grease. In a bowl, mix cucumber slices with spring onion, pepper flakes, vinegar, esame oil, sesame seeds, salt, pepper and noodles. Toss to coat well, keep in the fridge for 30 minutes and serve as a side for some grilled shrimp.

Nutrition: calories 400, fat 34, fiber 2, carbs 4, protein 2

Mixed Veggie Dish

Serve with a tasty keto steak!

Preparation time: 10 minutes
Cooking time: 10 minutes
Servings: 4
Ingredients:

- 14 ounces mushrooms, sliced
- 3 ounces broccoli florets
- 3.5 ounces sugar snap peas
- 6 tablespoons olive oil
- Salt and black pepper to the taste
- 3 ounces bell pepper, cut in strips
- 3 ounces spinach, torn
- 2 tablespoons garlic, minced
- 2 tablespoons pumpkin seeds
- A pinch of red pepper flakes

Directions:

Heat up a pan with the oil over medium high heat, add garlic, stir and cook for 1 minute. Add mushrooms, stir and cook fro 3 minutes more. Add broccoli and stir everything. Add snap peas and peppers and stir again. Add salt, pepper, pumpkin seeds and pepper flakes, stir and cook for a few minutes. Add spinach, stir gently, cook for a couple of minutes, divide on plates and serve as a side dish.

Nutrition: calories 247, fat 23, fiber 4, carbs 3, protein 7

Amazing Cauliflower Polenta

This should be very interesting! Let's learn how to prepare it!

Preparation time: 10 minutes
Cooking time: 1 hour
Servings: 2
Ingredients:

- 1 cauliflower head, florets separated
- ¼ cup hazelnuts
- 2 tablespoonы olive oil
- 1 small yellow onion, chopped
- 3 cups shiitake mushrooms, chopped
- 4 garlic cloves
- 3 tablespoons nutritional yeast
- ½ cup water
- Chopped parsley for serving

Directions:

Spread hazelnuts on a lined baking sheet, introduce in the oven at 350 degrees F and bake for 10 minutes. Take hazelnuts out of the oven, leave them to cool down, chop and leave aside for now. Spread cauliflower florets on the baking sheet, drizzle 1 teaspoon oil, introduce in the oven at 400 degrees F and bake for 30 minutes. In a bowl, mix oil with ½ teaspoon oil and toss to coat. Put garlic cloves on a tin foil, drizzle ½ teaspoon oil and wrap. Spread onion next to cauliflower, also add wrapped garlic to the baking sheet, introduce in the oven everything and bake for 20 minutes. Heat up a pan with the rest of the oil over medium high heat, add mushrooms, stir and cook for 8 minutes. Take cauliflower out of the oven and transfer to your food processor. Unwrap garlic, peel and also add to the food processor. Add onion, yeast, salt and pepper and blend everything well. Divide polenta on plates, top with mushrooms, hazelnuts and parsley and serve as a side.

Nutrition: calories 342, fat 21, fiber 12, carbs 3, protein 14

Amazing Side Dish
This will totally surprise you!

Preparation time: 10 minutes
Cooking time: 4 hours and 20 minutes
Servings: 8

Ingredients:

- 2 cups almond flour
- 2 tablespoons whey protein powder
- ¼ cup coconut flour
- ½ teaspoon garlic powder
- 2 teaspoons baking powder
- 1 and ¼ cups cheddar cheese, shredded
- 2 eggs
- ¼ cup melted ghee
- ¾ cup water

For the stuffing:
- ½ cup yellow onion, chopped
- 2 tablespoons ghee
- 1 red bell pepper, chopped
- 1 jalapeno pepper, chopped
- Salt and black pepper to the taste
- 12 ounces sausage, chopped
- 2 eggs
- ¾ cup chicken stock
- ¼ cup whipping cream

Directions:

In a bowl, mix coconut flour with whey protein, almond flour, garlic powder, baking powder and 1 cup cheddar cheese and stir everything. Add water, 2 eggs and ¼ cup ghee and stir well. Transfer this to a greased baking pan, sprinkle the rest of the cheddar cheese, introduce in the oven at 325 degrees F and bake for 30 minutes. Leave bread to cool down for 15 minutes and cube it. Spread bread cubes on a lined baking sheet, introduce in the oven at 200 degrees F and bake for 3 hours. Take bread cubes out of the oven and leave aside for now. Heat up a pan with 2 tablespoons ghee over medium heat, add onion, stir and cook for 4 minutes. Add jalapeno and red bell pepper, stir and cook for 5 minutes. Add salt and pepper, stir and transfer everything to a bowl. Heat up the same pan over medium heat, add sausage, stir and cook for 10 minutes. Transfer to the bowl with the veggies, also add stock, bread and stir everything. In a separate bowl, whisk 2 eggs with some salt, pepper and whipping cream. Add this over sausage and bread mix, stir, transfer to a greased baking pan, introduce in the oven at 325 degrees F and bake for 30 minutes. Serve hot as a side.

Nutrition: calories 340, fat 4, fiber 6, carbs 3.4, protein 7

Special Mushrooms

It's so yummy! You have to try it to see!

Preparation time: 10 minutes
Cooking time: 30 minutes
Servings: 4

Ingredients:

- 4 tablespoons ghee
- 16 ounces baby mushrooms
- Salt and black pepper to the taste
- 3 tablespoons onion, dried
- 3 tablespoons parsley flakes
- 1 teaspoon garlic powder

Directions:

In a bowl, mix parsley flakes with onion, salt, pepper and garlic powder and stir. In another bowl, mix mushroom with melted ghee and toss to coat. Add seasoning mix, toss well, spread on a lined baking sheet, introduce in the oven at 300 degrees F and bake for 30 minutes. Serve as a side dish for a tasty keto roast.

Nutrition: calories 152, fat 12, fiber 5, carbs 6, protein 4

Green Beans And Tasty Vinaigrette

You will find this keto side dish really amazing!

Preparation time: 10 minutes
Cooking time: 12 minutes
Serving: 8

Ingredients:

- 2 ounces chorizo, chopped
- 1 garlic clove, minced
- 1 teaspoon lemon juice
- 2 teaspoons smoked paprika
- ½ cup coconut vinegar
- 4 tablespoons macadamia nut oil
- ¼ teaspoon coriander, ground
- Salt and black pepper to the taste
- 2 tablespoons coconut oil
- 2 tablespoons beef stock
- 2 pound green beans

Directions:

In a blender, mix chorizo with salt, pepper, vinegar, garlic, lemon juice, paprika and coriander and pulse well. Add the stock and the macadamia nut oil and blend again. Heat up a pan with the coconut oil over medium heat, add green beans and chorizo mix, stir and cook for 10 minutes. Divide on plates and serve.

Nutrition: calories 160, fat 12, fiber 4, carbs 6, protein 4

Braised Eggplant Side Dish

Try this Vietnamese keto side dish!

Preparation time: 10 minutes
Cooking time: 15 minutes
Servings: 4
Ingredients:

- 1 big Asian eggplant, cut in medium pieces
- 1 yellow onion, thinly sliced
- 2 tablespoon vegetable oil
- 2 teaspoons garlic, minced
- ½ cu Vietnamese sauce
- ½ cup water
- 2 teaspoons chili paste
- ¼ cup coconut milk
- 4 green onions, chopped

For the Vietnamese sauce:

- 1 teaspoon palm sugar
- ½ cup chicken stock
- 2 tablespoons fish sauce

Directions:

Put stock in a pan and heat up over medium heat. Add sugar and fish sauce, stir well and leave aside for now. Heat up a pan over medium high heat, add eggplant pieces, brown them for 2 minutes and transfer to a plate. Heat up the pan again with the oil over medium high heat, add yellow onion and garlic, stir and cook for 2 minutes. Return eggplant pieces and cook for 2 minutes. Add water, the Vietnamese sauce you've made earlier, chili paste and coconut milk, stir and cook for 5 minutes. Add green onions, stir, cook for 1 minute more, transfer to plates and serve as a side dish.

Nutrition: calories 142, fat 7, fiber 4, carbs 5, protein 3

Cheddar Soufflés

If you are on a Ketogenic diet, then you must really try this side dish! Serve with a steak on the side!

Preparation time: 10 minutes
Cooking time: 25 minutes
Servings: 8
Ingredients:

- ¾ cup heavy cream
- 2 cups cheddar cheese, shredded
- 6 eggs
- Salt and black pepper to the taste
- ¼ teaspoon cream of tartar
- A pinch of cayenne pepper
- ½ teaspoon xanthan gum
- 1 teaspoon mustard powder
- ¼ cup chives, chopped
- ½ cup almond flour
- Cooking spray

Directions:

In a bowl, mix almond flour with salt, pepper, mustard, xantham gum and cayenne and whisk well. Add cheese, cream, chives, eggs and cream of tartar and whisk well again. Grease 8 ramekins with cooking spray, pour cheddar and chives mix, introduce in the oven at 350 degrees F and bake for 25 minutes. Serve your soufflés with a tasty keto steak.

Nutrition: calories 288, fat 23, fiber 1, carbs 3.3, protein 14

Tasty Cauliflower Side Salad
This is much better than you could ever imagine!

Preparation time: 10 minutes
Cooking time: 5 minutes
Servings: 10

Ingredients:

- 21 ounces cauliflower, florets separated
- Salt and black pepper to the taste
- 1 cup red onion, chopped
- 1 cup celery, chopped
- 2 tablespoons cider vinegar
- 1 teaspoon splenda
- 4 eggs, hard boiled, peeled and chopped
- 1 cup mayonnaise
- 1 tablespoon water

Directions:

Put cauliflower florets in a heat proof bowl, add the water, cover and cook in your microwave for 5 minutes. Leave aside for another 5 minutes and transfer to a salad bowl. Add celery, eggs and onions and stir gently. In a bowl, mix mayo with salt, pepper, splenda and vinegar and whisk well. Add this over salad, toss to coat well and serve right away as a side salad.

Nutrition: calories 211, fat 20, fiber 2, carbs 3, protein 4

Amazing Rice
Don't worry! It's not made with actual rice!

Preparation time: 10 minutes
Cooking time: 30 minutes
Servings: 4

Ingredients:

- 1 cauliflower head, florets separated
- Salt and black pepper to the taste
- 10 ounces coconut milk
- ½ cup water
- 2 ginger slices
- 2 tablespoons coconut shreds, toasted

Directions:

Put cauliflower in your food processor and blend. Transfer cauliflower rice to a kitchen towel, press well and leave aside. Heat up a pot with the coconut milk over medium heat. Add the water and ginger, stir and bring to a simmer. Add cauliflower, stir and cook for 30 minutes. Discard ginger, add salt, pepper and coconut shreds, stir gently, divide on plates and serve as a side for a poultry based dish.

Nutrition: calories 108, fat 3, fiber 6, carbs 5, protein 9

Ketogenic Snacks And Appetizers Recipes

Herbed Cheese Dip
It's a fact! These is delicious!

Preparation time: 10 minutes
Cooking time: 20 minutes
Servings: 4

Ingredients:

- A pinch of salt and black pepper
- 2 shallots, chopped
- 6 ounces cream cheese, soft
- 1 tablespoon cilantro, chopped
- 1 tablespoon chives, chopped

Directions:

In a bowl combine the cream cheese with the shallots and the other ingredients, whisk and divide into 4 ramekins. Introduce the ramekins in the oven, cook at 380 degrees F for 20 minutes and serve as a party dip.

Nutrition: calories 152, fat 14.9, fiber 0, carbs 2, protein 3.4

Cheesy Beef Dip
This is a great snack idea!

Preparation time: 10 minutes
Cooking time: 35 minutes
Servings: 6

Ingredients:

- 8 ounces cream cheese, soft
- A pinch of salt and black pepper
- 8 ounces beef stew meat, ground
- 2 shallots, chopped
- 2 tablespoons olive oil
- ¼ cup green onions, chopped

Directions:

Heat up a pan with the oil over medium heat, add the shallots and the green onions, stir and cook for 5 minutes. Add the meat and brown for 5 minutes more. Add the cream, salt and pepper, whisk, divide into 6 small ramekins, introduce them in the oven and cook at 380 degrees F for 25 minutes. Serve right away.

Nutrition: calories 246, fat 20.2, fiber 0.1, carbs 1.9, protein 14.5

Broccoli Dip

It's a really amazing combination! Try it!

Preparation time: 10 minutes
Cooking time: 30 minutes
Servings: 8
Ingredients:

- 1 cup heavy cream
- 1 pound broccoli florets
- 2 spring onions, chopped
- ¾ cup cream cheese
- ½ teaspoon chili powder
- 1 tablespoon chives, chopped

Directions:

In a pot, combine the cream with the broccoli and the other ingredients except the chives, stir, bring to a simmer over medium heat and cook for 30 minutes. Blend using an immersion blender, divide into bowls, sprinkle the chives on top and serve cold.

Nutrition: calories 149, fat 13.4, fiber 1.6, carbs 5.2, protein 3.6

Pesto Dip

It's one of the most tasty keto snacks ever!

Preparation time: 5 minutes
Cooking time: 0 minutes
Servings: 8
Ingredients:

- 2 cups basil
- 1 cup parmesan, grated
- 1 tablespoon pine nuts, toasted
- 2 tablespoons olive oil
- 1 garlic clove, minced
- A pinch of cayenne pepper

Directions:

In a blender, combine the basil with the other ingredients, pulse well, divide into small bowls and serve.

Nutrition: calories 73, fat 6.5, fiber 0.2, carbs 0.8, protein 3.7

Olives Dip

This snack is easy to make!

Preparation time: 10 minutes
Cooking time: 0 minutes
Servings: 4
Ingredients:

- 1 cup green olives, pitted and chopped
- 1 cup kalamata olives, pitted and chopped
- A pinch of salt and black pepper
- 2 tablespoons basil pesto
- 2 tablespoons olive oil
- ¼ cup cream cheese
- 1 tablespoons chives, chopped

Directions:

In a blender, combine the olives with the pesto and the other ingredients, pulse well, divide into small bowls and serve as a party dip.

Nutrition: calories 110, fat 10, fiber 0, carbs 1.4, protein 3

Zucchini Muffins
You can even take this snack at the office!

Preparation time: 10 minutes
Cooking time: 20 minutes
Servings: 6

Ingredients:
- ¼ cup coconut oil, melted
- 2 zucchinis, grated
- ¼ cup coconut flour
- ½ teaspoon nutmeg, ground
- ½ teaspoon baking soda
- 2 eggs, whisked
- ½ teaspoon baking powder
- A pinch of salt

Directions:
In a bowl, combine the zucchinis with the oil and the other ingredients and stir really well. Spoon this into a greased muffin pan, introduce in the oven at 370 degrees F and bake for 20 minutes. Leave muffins to cool down and serve them as a snack.

Nutrition: calories 131, fat 11.2, fiber 2.8, carbs 5.9, protein 3.3

Spinach Chips
It's an exceptional keto snack recipe!

Preparation time: 5 minutes
Cooking time: 15 minutes
Servings: 6

Ingredients:
- 1 tablespoon olive oil
- 1 pound baby spinach
- ½ teaspoon curry powder
- A pinch of salt and black pepper
- ½ teaspoon cumin, ground

Directions:
In a bowl, mix the spinach leaves with the oil and the other ingredients and toss gently. Spread the basil leaves well on a baking sheet lined with parchment paper, and cook in the oven at 420 degrees F for 15 minutes. Cool down and serve as a snack.

Nutrition: calories 30, fat 3, fiber 1.2, carbs 0.5, protein 1

Parsley Dip
This is flavored and delicious!

Preparation time: 5 minutes
Cooking time: 0 minutes
Servings: 6

Ingredients:
- 1 cup parsley
- 2 tablespoons pine nuts, toasted
- 2 tablespoons olive oil
- 3 ounces heavy cream
- ¼ teaspoon garlic powder
- A pinch of salt and black pepper
- 1 chili pepper, chopped

Directions:
In a blender, combine the parsley with the pine nuts and the other ingredients, pulse well, divide into small bowls and serve as a dip.

Nutrition: calories 130, fat 3.8, fiber 1, carbs 2.2, protein 5

Kale Muffins
This is a great keto appetizer!

Preparation time: 10 minutes
Cooking time: 30 minutes
Servings: 6

Ingredients:
- 1 cup almond flour
- Salt and black pepper to the taste
- 2 eggs
- 2 tablespoons coconut oil, melted
- 1 teaspoon baking powder
- 1 cup heavy cream
- 1 cup kale, chopped
- A pinch of salt and black pepper

Directions:
In a bowl, the flour with the eggs and the other ingredients, whisk well and divide into a muffin tray. Introduce in the oven at 350 degrees F, bake for 30 minutes and serve cold as a snack or appetizer.

Nutrition: calories 247, fat 22.3, fiber 2.2, carbs 6.2, protein 6.6

Cream Cheese Spread
You will love this great spread!

Preparation time: 10 minutes
Cooking time: 25 minutes
Servings: 4

Ingredients:
- 6 ounces cream cheese, soft
- ¼ cup parmesan, grated
- A pinch of salt and black pepper
- 1 tablespoon basil, chopped
- 1 tablespoon chives, chopped
- 1 teaspoon sweet paprika

Directions:
In a bowl, combine the cream cheese with the parmesan and the other ingredients, whisk well and divide into 4 ramekins. Introduce in the oven at 360 degrees F, bake for 25 minutes and serve cold.

Nutrition: calories 200, fat 5.4, fiber 4, carbs 5.4, protein 5.5

Beef Muffins
Everyone appreciates a great treat!

Preparation time: 10 minutes
Cooking time: 30 minutes
Servings: 6

Ingredients:
- ½ cup coconut flour
- 1 pound beef, ground and browned
- 2 eggs, whisked
- A pinch of salt and black pepper
- 2 spring onions, chopped
- Cooking spray
- ¼ teaspoon baking powder
- ¼ cup coconut milk

Directions:
In a bowl, combine the meat with the flour and the other ingredients except the cooking spray and stir well. Grease a muffin tray with the cooking spray, divide the beef mix in each muffin mould, introduce in the oven at 360 degrees F and bake for 30 minutes. Serve as an appetizer.

Nutrition: calories 227, fat 9.7, fiber 4.4, carbs 7.8, protein 26.4

Cheese and Leeks Dip

It's a tasty keto snack!

Preparation time: 10 minutes
Cooking time: 0 minutes
Servings: 4

Ingredients:

- 1 cup kalamata olives, pitted and chopped
- 6 ounces cream cheese, soft
- 1 tablespoon basil, chopped
- 1 tablespoon cilantro, chopped
- A pinch of red pepper flakes
- 2 tablespoons olive oil

Directions:

In a blender, combine the olives with the cream cheese and the other ingredients, pulse well, divide into small bowls and serve.

Nutrition: calories 247, fat 25.4, fiber 1.1, carbs 3.3, protein 3.5

Coconut Squares

This is a very healthy keto snack for you to try soon!

Preparation time: 10 minutes
Cooking time: 30 minutes
Servings: 8

Ingredients:

- 2 cups coconut flour
- 1 cup coconut flesh, unsweetened and shredded
- 1 cup walnuts, chopped
- 1 cup coconut oil
- ¼ teaspoon stevia
- Cooking spray

Directions:

In a bowl, combine the flour with the coconut flesh and the other ingredients except the cooking spray and stir well. Spread this in a baking dish greased with the cooking spray, press well on the bottom, introduce in the oven at 350 degrees F and bake for 30 minutes. Leave aside to cool down, cut into squares and serve.

Nutrition: calories 300, fat 13.4, fiber 1.2, carbs 6.2, protein 5

Herbs Spread

Try this herbed snack today!

Preparation time: 10 minutes
Cooking time: 0 minutes
Servings: 8

Ingredients:

- 1 cup cream cheese, soft
- ½ cup cheddar cheese, grated
- 2 tablespoons olive oil
- 2 tablespoons oregano, chopped
- 1 tablespoon chives, chopped
- 1 tablespoon rosemary, chopped
- 1 tablespoon parsley, chopped
- ¼ teaspoon garlic powder
- A pinch of salt and black pepper
- ¼ teaspoon sweet paprika

Directions:

In a blender, combine the cream cheese with the cheddar and the other ingredients, pulse well, divide into small bowls and serve.

Nutrition: calories 150, fat 6.3, fiber 1, carbs 5.1, protein 2

Thyme Leek Snack Bowls

These is a simple, yet very tasty keto snack!

Preparation time: 10 minutes
Cooking time: 30 minutes
Servings: 8

Ingredients:

- 2 tablespoons olive oil
- 3 leeks, sliced
- A pinch of salt and black pepper
- 2 teaspoons garlic, minced
- 1 tablespoon thyme, chopped
- 2 tablespoons parmesan, grated

Directions:

In a bowl, combine the leek slices with the oil and the other ingredients except the parmesan and toss. Spread the leeks on a baking sheet lined with parchment paper, sprinkle the cheese on top, introduce in the oven at 420 degrees F and bake for 30 minutes. Divide into bowls and serve as a snack.

Nutrition: calories 163, fat 13, fiber 1, carbs 5.3, protein 3

Cilantro and Leeks Dip

This is not a guacamole! It's much better

Preparation time: 10 minutes
Cooking time: 0 minutes
Servings: 4

Ingredients:

- ¼ cup cilantro, chopped
- 2 leeks, sliced
- Juice of 1 lime
- A pinch of salt and black pepper
- ½ cup coconut oil, melted
- ½ cup cream cheese, soft

Directions:

In a blender, combine the leeks with the cilantro and the other ingredients, pulse well, divide into small cups and serve as a party dip.!

Nutrition: calories 150, fat 14, fiber 2, carbs 4, protein 2

Shrimp Bowls

You've got to love this!

Preparation time: 10 minutes
Cooking time: 10 minutes
Servings: 6

Ingredients:

- 2 tablespoons olive oil
- 1 pound shrimp, peeled and deveined
- 1 tablespoons mint, chopped
- A pinch of salt and black pepper
- 1 teaspoon smoked paprika
- 1 cup baby spinach
- 1 avocado, peeled, pitted and cubed
- 1 tablespoon lime juice

Directions:

Spread the shrimp on a baking sheet lined with parchment paper, season with salt, pepper and the paprika, drizzle half of the oil, and bake at 400 degrees F for 10 minutes. Transfer the shrimp to a bowl, add the rest of the ingredients, toss, divide into smaller bowls and serve as an appetizer.

Nutrition: calories 245, fat 12, fiber 2, carbs 1, protein 14

Cheddar Cauliflower Bites

This snack will really make you feel full for a couple of hours!

Preparation time: 10 minutes
Cooking time: 25 minutes
Servings: 8

Ingredients:

- 1 pound cauliflower florets
- 1 teaspoon sweet paprika
- A pinch of salt and black pepper
- 2 eggs, whisked
- 1 cup coconut flour
- Cooking spray
- 1 cup cheddar cheese, grated

Directions:

In a bowl, mix the flour with salt, pepper, the cheese and the paprika and stir. Put the eggs in a separate bowl. Dredge the cauliflower florets in the eggs and then in the cheese mix, arrange them on a baking sheet lined with parchment paper and bake at 380 degrees F for 25 minutes. Serve as a snack.

Nutrition: calories 163, fat 12, fiber 2, carbs 2, protein 7

Turmeric Dip

These is so delicious and simple to make!

Preparation time: 10 minutes
Cooking time: 0 minutes
Servings: 4

Ingredients:

- 2 tablespoons olive oil
- 1 cup cream cheese, soft
- 1 teaspoon turmeric powder
- 1 tablespoon cilantro, chopped
- Salt and black pepper to the taste
- A pinch of cayenne pepper

Directions:

In a blender, combine the cream cheese with the turmeric and the other ingredients, pulse well, divide into small cups and serve.

Nutrition: calories 345, fat 33, fiber 4, carbs 5, protein 16

Stuffed Peppers
These look wonderful!

Preparation time: 10 minutes
Cooking time: 30 minutes
Servings: 4

Ingredients:
- 1 pound small bell peppers, halved
- A pinch of salt and black pepper
- 2 tablespoons olive oil
- 1 pound pork stew meat, ground
- 1 teaspoon sweet paprika
- ½ teaspoon rosemary, dried
- 1 cup mozzarella cheese, shredded
- 1 tablespoon chives, chopped

Directions:
Heat up a pan with the oil over medium heat, add the meat, salt and pepper, paprika and the rosemary, stir and brown for 10 minutes. Cool the mix down, add the eggs, whisk and stuff the peppers with this mix. Introduce in the oven at 400 degrees F, bake for 20 minutes and serve as an appetizer.

Nutrition: calories 350, fat 22, fiber 3, carbs 6, protein 27

Nuts and Seed Bowls
This is a great keto snack for a casual day!

Preparation time: 5 minutes
Cooking time: 20 minutes
Servings: 6

Ingredients:
- 1 cup walnuts
- 1 cup almonds
- 1 tablespoon sunflower seeds
- 2 tablespoons olive oil
- A pinch of salt and black pepper
- ½ teaspoon sweet paprika

Directions:
In a bowl, mix the walnuts with the almonds, seeds and the other ingredients, toss and spread on a baking sheet lined with parchment paper. Bake at 400 degrees F for 20 minutes, divide into bowls and serve as a snack.

Nutrition: calories 140, fat 2, fiber 1, carbs 5, protein 1

Tomato Dip
Try this today!

Preparation time: 10 minutes
Cooking time: 15 minutes
Servings: 4

Ingredients:
- 1 cup cream cheese, soft
- ¼ cup tomato passata
- 1 tablespoon basil, chopped
- ½ teaspoon sweet paprika
- Salt and black pepper to the taste

Directions:
In a bowl, combine the cream cheese with the passata and the other ingredients, whisk well, divide into 4 ramekins, introduce in the oven at 370 degrees F and bake for 15 minutes. Serve cold.

Nutrition: calories 140, fat 4, fiber 2, carbs 6, protein 4

Zucchini Salsa
Enjoy a great appetizer right away!

Preparation time: 10 minutes
Cooking time: 12 minutes
Servings: 6

Ingredients:
- 3 zucchinis, roughly cubed
- 3 spring onions, chopped
- 1 cup black olives, pitted and halved
- 1 cup cherry tomatoes, halved
- Salt and black pepper to the taste
- 2 tablespoons olive oil
- 2 tablespoons balsamic vinegar

Directions:
Heat up a pan with the oil over medium heat, add the spring onions and the zucchinis, stir and sauté for 2 minutes. Add the rest of the ingredients, toss, cook for 10 minutes more, divide into bowls and serve cold.

Nutrition: calories 40, fat 3, fiber 7, carbs 3, protein 7

Leeks Hummus

Everyone loves a good hummus! Try this one!

Preparation time: 5 minutes
Cooking time: 0 minutes
Servings: 4

Ingredients:
- 4 leeks, chopped
- ¼ cup avocado oil
- Salt and black pepper to the taste
- 4 garlic cloves, minced
- 1 cup sesame seeds paste
- 2 tablespoons lime juice
- 1 tablespoon chives, chopped

Directions:

In your blender, mix the leeks with the oil, salt, pepper and the other ingredients, pulse well, divide into bowls and serve cold.

Nutrition: calories 80, fat 5, fiber 3, carbs 6, protein 7

Chicken Dip

This is so great!

Preparation time: 6 minutes
Cooking time: 0 minutes
Servings: 8

Ingredients:
- 2 cups rotisserie chicken, skinless, boneless shredded
- 2 red chilies, minced
- 2 spring onions, chopped
- ¼ cup cream cheese, soft
- Salt and black pepper to the taste
- ½ teaspoon smoked paprika

Directions:

In a bowl, combine the chicken with the chilies and the other ingredients, stir well, divide into small bowls and serve as a party dip.

Nutrition: calories 100, fat 2, fiber 3, carbs 1, protein 6

Beef Jerky Snack
We are sure you will love this keto snack!

Preparation time: 6 hours
Cooking time: 4 hours
Servings: 6

Ingredients:
- 24 ounces amber
- 2 cups soy sauce
- ½ cup Worcestershire sauce
- 2 tablespoons black peppercorns
- 2 tablespoons black pepper
- 2 pounds beef round, sliced

Directions:
In a bowl, mix soy sauce with black peppercorns, black pepper and Worcestershire sauce and whisk well. Add beef slices, toss to coat and leave aside in the fridge for 6 hours. Spread this on a rack, introduce in the oven at 370 degrees F and bake for 4 hours. Transfer to a bowl and serve.

Nutrition: calories 300, fat 12, fiber 4, carbs 3, protein 8

Crab Dip
You will adore this amazing keto appetizer!

Preparation time: 10 minutes
Cooking time: 30 minutes
Servings: 8

Ingredients:
- 8 bacon strips, sliced
- 12 ounces crab meat
- ½ cup mayonnaise
- ½ cup sour cream
- 8 ounces cream cheese
- 2 poblano pepper, chopped
- 2 tablespoons lemon juice
- Salt and black pepper to the taste
- 4 garlic cloves, minced
- 4 green onions, minced
- ½ cup parmesan cheese+ ½ cup parmesan cheese, grated
- Salt and black pepper to the taste

Directions:
Heat up a pan over medium high heat, add bacon, cook until it's crispy, transfer to paper towels, chop and leave aside to cool down. In a bowl, mix sour cream with cream cheese and mayo and stir well. Add ½ cup parmesan, poblano peppers, bacon, green onion, garlic and lemon juice and stir again. Add crab meat, salt and pepper and stir gently. Pour this into a heat proof baking dish, spread the rest of the parmesan, introduce in the oven and bake at 350 degrees F for 20 minutes. Serve your dip warm with cucumber stick.

Nutrition: calories 200, fat 7, fiber 2, carbs 4, protein 6

Simple Spinach Balls

This is a very tasty keto party appetizer!

Preparation time: 10 minutes
Cooking time: 12 minutes
Servings: 30
Ingredients:

- 4 tablespoons melted ghee
- 2 eggs
- 1 cup almond flour
- 16 ounces spinach
- 1/3 cup feta cheese, crumbled
- ¼ teaspoon nutmeg, ground
- 1/3 cup parmesan, grated
- Salt and black pepper to the taste
- 1 tablespoon onion powder
- 3 tablespoons whipping cream
- 1 teaspoon garlic powder

Directions:

In your blender, mix spinach with ghee, eggs, almond flour, feta cheese, parmesan, nutmeg, whipping cream, salt, pepper, onion and garlic pepper and blend very well. Transfer to a bowl and keep in the freezer for 10 minutes Shape 30 spinach balls, arrange on a lined baking sheet, introduce in the oven at 350 degrees F and bake for 12 minutes. Leave spinach balls to cool down and serve as a party appetizer.

Nutrition: calories 60, fat 5, fiber 1, carbs 0.7, protein 2

Garlic Spinach Dip

This keto appetizer will make you love spinach even more!

Preparation time: 10 minutes
Cooking time: 35 minutes
Servings: 6
Ingredients:

- 6 bacon slices
- 5 ounces spinach
- ½ cup sour cream
- 8 ounces cream cheese, soft
- 1 and ½ tablespoons parsley, chopped
- 2.5 ounces parmesan, grated
- 1 tablespoon lemon juice
- Salt and black pepper to the taste
- 1 tablespoon garlic, minced

Directions:

Heat up a pan over medium heat, add bacon, cook until it's crispy, transfer to paper towels, drain grease, crumble and leave aside in a bowl. Heat up the same pan with the bacon grease over medium heat, add spinach, stir, cook for 2 minutes and transfer to a bowl. In another bowl, mix cream cheese with garlic, salt, pepper, sour cream and parsley and stir well. Add bacon and stir again. Add lemon juice and spinach and stir everything. Add parmesan and stir again. Divide this into ramekins, introduce in the oven at 350 degrees f and bake for 25 minutes. Turn oven to broil and broil for 4 minutes more. Serve with crackers.

Nutrition: calories 345, fat 12, fiber 3, carbs 6, protein 11

Mushrooms Appetizer
These mushrooms are so yummy!

Preparation time: 10 minutes
Cooking time: 20 minutes
Servings: 5

Ingredients:
- ¼ cup mayo
- 1 teaspoon garlic powder
- 1 small yellow onion, chopped
- 24 ounces white mushroom caps
- Salt and black pepper to the taste
- 1 teaspoon curry powder
- 4 ounces cream cheese, soft
- ¼ cup sour cream
- ½ cup Mexican cheese, shredded
- 1 cup shrimp, cooked, peeled, deveined and chopped

Directions:
In a bowl, mix mayo with garlic powder, onion, curry powder, cream cheese, sour cream, Mexican cheese, shrimp, salt and pepper to the taste and whisk well. Stuff mushrooms with this mix, place on a baking sheet and cook in the oven at 350 degrees F for 20 minutes. Arrange on a platter and serve.

Nutrition: calories 244, fat 20, fiber 3, carbs 7, protein 14

Simple Bread Sticks
You just have to give this amazing keto snack a chance!

Preparation time: 10 minutes
Cooking time: 15 minutes
Servings: 24

Ingredients:
- 3 tablespoons cream cheese, soft
- 1 tablespoon psyllium powder
- ¾ cup almond flour
- 2 cups mozzarella cheese, melted for 30 seconds in the microwave
- 1 teaspoon baking powder
- 1 egg
- 2 tablespoons Italian seasoning
- Salt and black pepper to the taste
- 3 ounces cheddar cheese, grated
- 1 teaspoon onion powder

Directions:
In a bowl, mix psyllium powder with almond flour, baking powder, salt and pepper and whisk. Add cream cheese, melted mozzarella and egg and stir using your hands until you obtain a dough. Spread this on a baking sheet and cut into 24 sticks. Sprinkle onion powder and Italian seasoning over them. Top with cheddar cheese, introduce in the oven at 350 degrees F and bake for 15 minutes. Serve them as a keto snack!

Nutrition: calories 245, fat 12, fiber 5, carbs 3, protein 14

Italian Meatballs
This Italian style appetizer is 100% keto!

Preparation time: 10 minutes
Cooking time: 6 minutes
Servings: 16

Ingredients:
- 1 egg
- Salt and black pepper to the taste
- ¼ cup almond flour
- 1 pound turkey meat, ground
- ½ teaspoon garlic powder
- 2 tablespoons sun dried tomatoes, chopped
- ½ cup mozzarella cheese, shredded
- 2 tablespoons olive oil
- 2 tablespoon basil, chopped

Directions:
In a bowl, mix turkey with salt, pepper, egg, almond flour, garlic powder, sun dried tomatoes, mozzarella and basil and stir well. Shape 12 meatballs, heat up a pan with the oil over medium high heat, drop meatballs and cook them for 2 minutes on each side. Arrange on a platter and serve.

Nutrition: calories 80, fat 6, fiber 3, carbs 5, protein 7

Parmesan Wings
These will be appreciated by all your family!

Preparation time: 10 minutes
Cooking time: 24 minutes
Servings: 6

Ingredients:
- 6 pound chicken wings, cut in halves
- Salt and black pepper to the taste
- ½ teaspoon Italian seasoning
- 2 tablespoons ghee
- ½ cup parmesan cheese, grated
- A pinch of red pepper flakes, crushed
- 1 teaspoon garlic powder
- 1 egg

Directions:
Arrange chicken wings on a lined baking sheet, introduce in the oven at 425 degrees F and bake for 17 minutes. Meanwhile, in your blender, mix ghee with cheese, egg, salt, pepper, pepper flakes, garlic powder and Italian seasoning and blend very well. Take chicken wings out of the oven, flip them, turn oven to broil and broil them for 5 minutes more. Take chicken pieces out of the oven again, pour sauce over them, toss to coat well and broil for 1 minute more. Serve them as a quick keto appetizer.

Nutrition: calories 134, fat 8, fiber 1, carbs 0.5, protein 14

Cheese Sticks

This keto appetizer will simply melt into your mouth!

Preparation time: 1 hour and 10 minutes
Cooking time: 20 minutes
Servings: 16

Ingredients:

- 2 eggs, whisked
- Salt and black pepper to the taste
- 8 mozzarella cheese strings, cut in halves
- 1 cup parmesan, grated
- 1 tablespoon Italian seasoning
- ½ cup olive oil
- 1 garlic clove, minced

Directions:

In a bowl, mix parmesan with salt, pepper, Italian seasoning and garlic and stir well. Put whisked eggs in another bowl. Dip mozzarella sticks in egg mixture, then in cheese mix. Dip them again in egg and in the parmesan mix and keep them in the freezer for 1 hour. Heat up a pan with the oil over medium high heat, add cheese sticks, fry them until they are golden on one side, flip and cook them the same way on the other side. Arrange them on a platter and serve.

Nutrition: calories 140, fat 5, fiber 1, carbs 3, protein 4

Tasty Broccoli Sticks

You must invite all your friends to taste this keto appetizer!

Preparation time: 10 minutes
Cooking time: 20 minutes
Servings: 20

Ingredients:

- 1 egg
- 2 cups broccoli florets
- 1/3 cup cheddar cheese, grated
- ¼ cup yellow onion, chopped
- 1/3 cup panko breadcrumbs
- 1/3 cup Italian breadcrumbs
- 2 tablespoons parsley, chopped
- A drizzle of olive oil
- Salt and black pepper to the taste

Directions:

Heat up a pot with water over medium heat, add broccoli, steam for 1 minute, drain, chop and put into a bowl. Add egg, cheddar cheese, panko and Italian breadcrumbs, salt, pepper and parsley and stir everything well. Shape sticks out of this mix using your hands and place them on a baking sheet which you've greased with some olive oil. Introduce in the oven at 400 degrees F and bake for 20 minutes. Arrange on a platter and serve.

Nutrition: calories 100, fat 4, fiber 2, carbs 7, protein 7

Bacon Delight

Don't be afraid to try this special and very tasty keto snack!

Preparation time: 15 minutes
Cooking time: 1 hour and 20 minutes
Servings: 16

Ingredients:
- ½ teaspoon cinnamon, ground
- 2 tablespoons erythritol
- 16 bacon slices
- 1 tablespoon coconut oil
- 3 ounces dark chocolate
- 1 teaspoon maple extract

Directions:
In a bowl, mix cinnamon with erythritol and stir. Arrange bacon slices on a lined baking sheet and sprinkle cinnamon mix over them. Flip bacon slices and sprinkle cinnamon mix over them again. Introduce in the oven at 275 degrees F and bake for 1 hour. Heat up a pot with the oil over medium heat, add chocolate and stir until it melts. Add maple extract, stir, take off heat and leave aside to cool down a bit. Take bacon strips out of the oven, leave them to cool down, dip each in chocolate mix, place them on a parchment paper and leave them to cool down completely. Serve cold.

Nutrition: calories 150, fat 4, fiber 0.4, carbs 1.1, protein 3

Taco Cups

These taco cups make the perfect party appetizer!

Preparation time: 10 minutes
Cooking time: 40 minutes
Servings: 30

Ingredients:
- 1 pound beef, ground
- 2 cups cheddar cheese, shredded
- ¼ cup water
- Salt and black pepper to the taste
- 2 tablespoons cumin
- 2 tablespoons chili powder
- Pico de gallo for serving

Directions:
Divide spoonfuls of parmesan on a lined baking sheet, introduce in the oven at 350 degrees F and bake for 7 minutes. Leave cheese to cool down for 1 minute, transfer them to mini cupcake molds and shape them into cups. Meanwhile, heat up a pan over medium high heat, add beef, stir and cook until it browns. Add the water, salt, pepper, cumin and chili powder, stir and cook for 5 minutes more. Divide into cheese cups, top with pico de gallo, transfer them all to a platter and serve.

Nutrition: calories 140, fat 6, fiber 0, carbs 6, protein 15

Tasty Chicken Egg Rolls
These are just what you need! It's the best keto party appetizer!

Preparation time: 2 hours and 10 minutes
Cooking time: 15 minutes
Servings: 12

Ingredients:

- 4 ounces blue cheese
- 2 cups chicken, cooked and finely chopped
- Salt and black pepper to the taste
- 2 green onions, chopped
- 2 celery stalks, finely chopped
- ½ cup tomato sauce
- ½ teaspoon erythritol
- 12 egg roll wrappers
- Vegetable oil

Directions:

In a bowl, mix chicken meat with blue cheese, salt, pepper, green onions, celery, tomato sauce and sweetener, stir well and keep in the fridge for 2 hours. Place egg wrappers on a working surface, divide chicken mix on them, roll and seal edges. Heat up a pan with vegetable oil over medium high heat, add egg rolls, cook until they are golden, flip and cook on the other side as well. Arrange on a platter and serve them.

Nutrition: calories 220, fat 7, fiber 2, carbs 6, protein 10

Halloumi Cheese Fries
These are so crunchy and delightful!

Preparation time: 10 minutes
Cooking time: 5 minutes
Servings: 4

Ingredients:

- 1 cup marinara sauce
- 8 ounces halloumi cheese, pat dried and sliced into fries
- 2 ounces tallow

Directions:

Heat up a pan with the tallow over medium high heat. Add halloumi pieces, cover, cook for 2 minutes on each side and transfer to paper towels. Drain excess grease, transfer them to a bowl and serve with marinara sauce on the side.

Nutrition: calories 200, fat 16, fiber 1, carbs 1, protein 13

Jalapeno Crisps

These are so easy to make at home!

Preparation time: 10 minutes
Cooking time: 25 minutes
Servings: 20

Ingredients:
- 3 tablespoons olive oil
- 5 jalapenos, sliced
- 8 ounces parmesan cheese, grated
- ½ teaspoon onion powder
- Salt and black pepper to the taste
- Tabasco sauce for serving

Directions:
In a bowl, mix jalapeno slices with salt, pepper, oil and onion powder, toss to coat and spread on a lined baking sheet. Introduce in the oven at 450 degrees F and bake for 15 minutes. Take jalapeno slices out of the oven, leave them to cool down. In a bowl, mix pepper slices with the cheese and press well. Arrange all slices on a another lined baking sheet, introduce in the oven again and bake for 10 minutes more. Leave jalapenos to cool down, arrange on a plate and serve with Tabasco sauce on the side.

Nutrition: calories 50, fat 3, fiber 0.1, carbs 0.3, protein 2

Delicious Cucumber Cups

Get ready to taste something really elegant and delicious!

Preparation time: 10 minutes
Cooking time: 0 minutes
Servings: 24

Ingredients:
- 2 cucumbers, peeled, cut in ¾ inch slices and some of the seeds scooped out
- ½ cup sour cream
- Salt and white pepper to the taste
- 6 ounces smoked salmon, flaked
- 1/3 cup cilantro, chopped
- 2 teaspoons lime juice
- 1 tablespoon lime zest
- A pinch of cayenne pepper

Directions:
In a bowl mix salmon with salt, pepper, cayenne, sour cream, lime juice and zest and cilantro and stir well. Fill each cucumber cup with this salmon mix, arrange on a platter and serve as a keto appetizer.

Nutrition: calories 30, fat 11, fiber 1, carbs 1, protein 2

Caviar Salad

This is so elegant! It's so delicious and sophisticated!

Preparation time: 6 minutes
Cooking time: 0 minutes
Servings: 16

Ingredients:

- 8 eggs, hard boiled, peeled and mashed with a fork
- 4 ounces black caviar
- 4 ounces red caviar
- Salt and black pepper to the taste
- 1 yellow onion, finely chopped
- ¾ cup mayonnaise
- Some toast baguette slices for serving

Directions:

In a bowl, mix mashed eggs with mayo, salt, pepper and onion and stir well. Spread eggs salad on toasted baguette slices, and top each with caviar.

Nutrition: calories 122, fat 8, fiber 1, carbs 4, protein 7

Marinated Kebabs

This is the perfect appetizer for a summer barbeque!

Preparation time: 20 minutes
Cooking time: 10 minutes
Servings: 6

Ingredients:

- 1 red bell pepper, cut in chunks
- 1 green bell pepper, cut into chunks
- 1 orange bell pepper, cut into chunks
- 2 pounds sirloin steak, cut into medium cubes
- 4 garlic cloves, minced
- 1 red onion, cut into chunks
- Salt and black pepper to the taste
- 2 tablespoons Dijon mustard
- 2 and ½ tablespoons Worcestershire sauce
- ¼ cup tamari sauce
- ¼ cup lemon juice
- ½ cup olive oil

Directions:

In a bowl, mix Worcestershire sauce with salt, pepper, garlic, mustard, tamari, lemon juice and oil and whisk very well. Add beef, bell peppers and onion chunks to this mix, toss to coat and leave aside for a few minutes. Arrange bell pepper, meat cubes and onion chunks on skewers alternating colors, place them on your preheated grill over medium high heat, cook for 5 minutes on each side, transfer to a platter and serve as a summer keto appetizer.

Nutrition: calories 246, fat 12, fiber 1, carbs 4, protein 26

Simple Zucchini Rolls

You've got to try this simple and very tasty appetizer as soon as possible!

Preparation time: 10 minutes
Cooking time: 5 minutes
Servings: 24

Ingredients:

- 2 tablespoons olive oil
- 3 zucchinis, thinly sliced
- 24 basil leaves
- 2 tablespoons mint, chopped
- 1 and 1/3 cup ricotta cheese
- Salt and black pepper to the taste
- ¼ cup basil, chopped
- Tomato sauce for serving

Directions:

Brush zucchini slices with the olive oil, season with salt and pepper on both sides, place them on preheated grill over medium heat, cook them for 2 minutes, flip and cook for another 2 minutes. Place zucchini slices on a plate and leave aside for now. In a bowl, mix ricotta with chopped basil, mint, salt and pepper and stir well. Spread this over zucchini slices, divide whole basil leaves as well, roll and serve as an appetizer with some tomato sauce on the side.

Nutrition: calories 40, fat 3, fiber 0.3, carbs 1, protein 2

Simple Green Crackers

These are real fun to make and they taste amazing!

Preparation time: 10 minutes
Cooking time: 24 hours
Servings: 6

Ingredients:

- 2 cups flax seed, ground
- 2 cups flax seed, soaked overnight and drained
- 4 bunches kale, chopped
- 1 bunch basil, chopped
- ½ bunch celery, chopped
- 4 garlic cloves, minced
- 1/3 cup olive oil

Directions:

In your food processor mix ground flaxseed with celery, kale, basil and garlic and blend well. Add oil and soaked flaxseed and blend again. Spread this into a tray, cut into medium crackers, introduce in your dehydrator and dry for 24 hours at 115 degrees F, turning them halfway. Arrange them on a platter and serve.

Nutrition: calories 100, fat 1, fiber 2, carbs 1, protein 4

Cheese And Pesto Terrine

This looks so amazing and it tastes great!

Preparation time: 30 minutes
Cooking time: 0 minutes
Servings: 10
Ingredients:

- ½ cup heavy cream
- 10 ounces goat cheese, crumbled
- 3 tablespoons basil pesto
- 5 sun dried tomatoes, chopped
- ¼ cup pine nuts, toasted and
- 1 tablespoons pine nuts

Directions:

In a bowl, mix goat cheese with the heavy cream, salt and pepper and stir using your mixer. Spoon half of this mix into a lined bowl and spread. Add pesto on top and also spread. Add another layer of cheese, then add sun dried tomatoes and ¼ cup pine nuts. Spread one last layer of cheese and top with 1 tablespoon pine nuts. Keep in the fridge for a while, turn upside down on a plate and serve.
Nutrition: calories 240, fat 12, fiber 3, carbs 5, protein 12

Avocado Salsa

You will make this over and over again! That's how tasty it is!

Preparation time: 10 minutes
Cooking time: 0 minutes
Servings: 4
Ingredients:

- 1 small red onion, chopped
- 2 avocados, pitted, peeled and chopped
- 3 jalapeno pepper, chopped
- Salt and black pepper to the taste
- 2 tablespoons cumin powder
- 2 tablespoons lime juice
- ½ tomato, chopped

Directions:

In a bowl, mix onion with avocados, peppers, salt, black pepper, cumin, lime juice and tomato pieces and stir well. Transfer this to a bowl and serve with toasted baguette slices as a keto appetizer.
Nutrition: calories 120, fat 2, fiber 2, carbs 0.4, protein 4

Tasty Egg Chips

Do you want to impress everyone? Then, try these chips!

Preparation time: 5 minutes
Cooking time: 10 minutes
Servings: 2
Ingredients:

- ½ tablespoon water
- 2 tablespoons parmesan, shredded
- 4 eggs whites
- Salt and black pepper to the taste

Directions:

In a bowl, mix egg whites with salt, pepper and water and whisk well. Spoon this into a muffin pan, sprinkle cheese on top, introduce in the oven at 400 degrees F and bake for 15 minutes. Transfer egg white chips to a platter and serve with a keto dip on the side.
Nutrition: calories 120, fat 2, fiber 1, carbs 2, protein 7

Chili Lime Chips

These crackers will impress you with their amazing taste!

Preparation time: 10 minutes
Cooking time: 20 minutes
Servings: 4

Ingredients:
- 1 cup almond flour
- 1 and ½ teaspoons lime zest
- 1 teaspoon lime juice
- 1 egg

Directions:
In a bowl, mix almond flour with lime zest, lime juice and salt and stir. Add egg and whisk well again. Divide this into 4 parts, roll each into a ball and then spread well using a rolling pin. Cut each into 6 triangles, place them all on a lined baking sheet, introduce in the oven at 350 degrees F and bake for 20 minutes.

Nutrition: calories 90, fat 1, fiber 1, carbs 0.6, protein 3

Artichoke Dip

It's so rich and flavored!

Preparation time: 10 minutes
Cooking time: 15 minutes
Servings: 16

Ingredients:
- ¼ cup sour cream
- ¼ cup heavy cream
- ¼ cup mayonnaise
- ¼ cup shallot, chopped
- 1 tablespoon olive oil
- 2 garlic cloves, minced
- 4 ounces cream cheese
- ½ cup parmesan cheese, grated
- 1 cup mozzarella cheese, shredded
- 4 ounces feta cheese, crumbled
- 1 tablespoon balsamic vinegar
- 28 ounces canned artichoke hearts, chopped
- Salt and black pepper to the taste
- 10 ounces spinach, chopped

Directions:
Heat up a pan with the oil over medium heat, add shallot and garlic, stir and cook for 3 minutes. Add heavy cream and cream cheese and stir. Also add sour cream, parmesan, mayo, feta cheese and mozzarella cheese, stir and reduce heat. Add artichoke, spinach, salt, pepper and vinegar, stir well, take off heat and transfer to a bowl.

Nutrition: calories 144, fat 12, fiber 2, carbs 5, protein 5

Ketogenic Fish And Seafood Recipes

Creamy Mackerel
This is really creamy and rich!

Preparation time: 10 minutes
Cooking time: 20 minutes
Servings: 4

Ingredients:

- 2 shallots, minced
- 2 spring onions, chopped
- 2 tablespoons olive oil
- 4 mackerel fillets, skinless and cut into medium cubes
- 1 cup heavy cream
- 1 teaspoon cumin, ground
- ½ teaspoon oregano, dried
- A pinch of salt and black pepper
- 2 tablespoons chives, chopped

Directions:
Heat up a pan with the oil over medium heat, add the spring onions and the shallots, stir and sauté for 5 minutes. Add the fish and cook it for 4 minutes. Add the rest of the ingredients, bring to a simmer, cook everything for 10 minutes more, divide between plates and serve.

Nutrition: calories 403, fat 33.9, fiber 0.4, carbs 2.7, protein 22

Lime Mackerel
It's an easy keto dish for you to enjoy tonight for dinner!

Preparation time: 10 minutes
Cooking time: 30 minutes
Servings: 4

Ingredients:

- 4 mackerel fillets, boneless
- 2 tablespoons lime juice
- 2 tablespoons olive oil
- A pinch of salt and black pepper
- ½ teaspoon sweet paprika

Directions:
Arrange the mackerel on a baking sheet lined with parchment paper, add the oil and the other ingredients, rub gently, introduce in the oven at 360 degrees F and bake for 30 minutes. Divide the fish between plates and serve.

Nutrition: calories 297, fat 22.7, fiber 0.2, carbs 2, protein 21.1

Turmeric Tilapia
This great dish is perfect for a special evening!

Preparation time: 10 minutes
Cooking time: 12 minutes
Servings: 4

Ingredients:

- 4 tilapia fillets, boneless
- 2 tablespoons olive oil
- 1 teaspoon turmeric powder
- A pinch of salt and black pepper
- 2 spring onions, chopped
- ¼ teaspoon basil, dried
- ¼ teaspoon garlic powder
- 1 tablespoon parsley, chopped

Directions:

Heat up a pan with the oil over medium heat, add the spring onions and cook them for 2 minutes. Add the fish, turmeric and the other ingredients, cook for 5 minutes on each side, divide between plates and serve.

Nutrition: calories 205, fat 8.6, fiber 0.4, carbs 1.1, protein 31.8

Walnut Salmon Mix
You just have to try this wonderful combination!

Preparation time: 10 minutes
Cooking time: 14 minutes
Servings: 4

Ingredients:

- 4 salmon fillets, boneless
- 2 tablespoons avocado oil
- A pinch of salt and black pepper
- 1 tablespoon lime juice
- 2 shallots, chopped
- 2 tablespoons walnuts, chopped
- 2 tablespoons parsley, chopped

Directions:

Heat up a pan with the oil over medium high heat, add the shallots, stir and sauté for 2 minutes. Add the fish and the other ingredients, cook for 6 minutes on each side, divide between plates and serve.

Nutrition: calories 276, fat 14.2, fiber 0.7, carbs 2.7, protein 35.8

Chives Trout

The fish is so rich and flavored!

Preparation time: 10 minutes
Cooking time: 12 minutes
Servings: 4

Ingredients:
- 4 trout fillets, boneless
- 2 shallots, chopped
- A pinch of salt and black pepper
- 3 tablespoons chives, chopped
- 2 tablespoons avocado oil
- 2 teaspoons lime juice

Directions:
Heat up a pan with the oil over medium heat, add the shallots and sauté them for 2 minutes. Add the fish and the rest of the ingredients, cook for 5 minutes on each side, divide between plate sand serve.

Nutrition: calories 320, fat 12, fiber 1, carbs 2, protein 24

Salmon and Tomatoes

Feel free to serve this great dish today1

Preparation time: 10 minutes
Cooking time: 25 minutes
Servings: 4

Ingredients:
- 2 tablespoons avocado oil
- 4 salmon fillets, boneless
- 1 cup cherry tomatoes, halved
- 2 spring onions, chopped
- ½ cup chicken stock
- A pinch of salt and black pepper
- ½ teaspoon rosemary, dried

Directions:
In a roasting pan, combine the fish with the oil and the other ingredients, introduce in the oven at 400 degrees F and bake for 25 minutes. Divide between plates and serve.

Nutrition: calories 200, fat 12, fiber 0, carbs 3, protein 21

Trout and Mustard Sauce

Enjoy this flavored fish and sauce!

Preparation time: 5 minutes
Cooking time: 20 minutes
Servings: 4

Ingredients:

- 2 tablespoons olive oil
- 2 garlic cloves, minced
- 2 spring onions, chopped
- 4 trout fillets, boneless
- A pinch of salt and black pepper
- 2 tablespoons Dijon mustard
- Juice and zest of 1 lime
- ½ cup heavy cream
- 2 tablespoons chives, chopped

Directions:

Heat up a pan with the oil over medium heat, add the garlic and the spring onions, stir and sauté for 3 minutes. Add the fish and the cook it for 4 minutes on each side. Add the mustard and the other ingredients, toss gently, cook over medium heat for 10 minutes more, divide between plates and serve.

Nutrition: calories 171, fat 5, fiber 1, carbs 6, protein 23

Sea Bass and Olives

This dish is wonderful and very simple to make!

Preparation time: 10 minutes
Cooking time: 20 minutes
Servings: 4

Ingredients:

- 4 sea bass fillets, boneless
- 2 tablespoons avocado oil
- A pinch of salt and black pepper
- 1 cup kalamata olives, pitted and sliced
- 1 tablespoon oregano, chopped
- 2 tablespoons capers, drained
- 1 tablespoon lime juice
- 1 tablespoon cilantro, chopped

Directions:

Heat up a pan with the oil over medium heat, add the fish and cook it for 4 minutes on each side. Add the olives and the other ingredients, toss gently, cook over medium-low heat for 10 minutes more, divide between plates and serve.

Nutrition: calories 245, fat 12, fiber 1, carbs 3, protein 23

Paprika Shrimp Mix

This is so juicy and delicious!

Preparation time: 10 minutes
Cooking time: 10 minutes
Servings: 4

Ingredients:

- 1 pound shrimp, peeled and deveined
- 3 garlic cloves, minced
- 2 shallots, minced
- 2 tablespoons olive oil
- Juice of 1 lime
- 2 teaspoons sweet paprika
- 2 tablespoons parsley, chopped

Directions:

Heat up a pan with the oil over medium heat, add the garlic and the shallots, stir and cook for 2 minutes. Add the shrimp and the other ingredients, cook over medium heat for 8 minutes more, divide between plates and serve.

Nutrition: calories 205, fat 9.1, fiber 0.6, carbs 4.1, protein 26.2

Hot Shrimp Mix

This is the best shrimp mix!

Preparation time: 10 minutes
Cooking time: 10 minutes
Servings: 4

Ingredients:

- 1 pound shrimp, peeled and deveined
- 2 tablespoons green onions, chopped
- 2 tablespoons olive oil
- 2 red chilies, chopped
- ½ teaspoon hot paprika
- ¼ cup chicken stock
- 1 tablespoon chives, chopped

Directions:

Heat up a pan with the oil over medium heat, add the green onions and the chilies, stir and cook for 2 minutes. Add the shrimp and the other ingredients, cook over medium heat for 8 minutes more, divide into bowls and serve.

Nutrition: calories 197, fat 9, fiber 0.1, carbs 2, protein 25.9

Garlic Calamari Mix
The crust is wonderful!

Preparation time: 10 minutes
Cooking time: 25 minutes
Servings: 4

Ingredients:

- 3 garlic cloves, minced
- 2 tablespoons olive oil
- 1 pound calamari rings
- 1 tablespoon balsamic vinegar
- 1 cup chicken stock
- A pinch of salt and black pepper
- ¼ cup parsley, chopped

Directions:

Heat up a pan with the oil over medium heat, add the garlic, stir and cook for 5 minutes. Add the calamari and the other ingredients, toss, bring to a simmer and cook over medium heat for 20 minutes. Divide the mix into bowls and serve.

Nutrition: calories 240, fat 12, fiber 6.1, carbs 5.6, protein 25

Cod and Zucchinis
It's perfect keto dish for a weekend meal!

Preparation time: 10 minutes
Cooking time: 20 minutes
Servings: 4

Ingredients:

- 4 cod fillets, boneless
- 2 tablespoons olive oil
- 2 zucchinis, cubed
- 2 shallots, chopped
- 1 tomato, cubed
- ½ cup chicken stock
- ½ teaspoon sweet paprika
- A pinch of salt and black pepper
- 1 tablespoon cilantro, chopped

Directions:

Heat up a pan with the oil over medium heat, add the shallots, stir and cook for 2 minutes. Add the fish, and cook it for 4 minutes on each side. Add the rest of the ingredients, cook over medium heat for 10 minutes more, divide between plates and serve.

Nutrition: calories 200, fat 6, fiber 1, carbs 4, protein 20

Cumin Salmon
This grilled salmon is so awesome!

Preparation time: 10 minutes
Cooking time: 10 minutes
Servings: 4

Ingredients:

- 4 salmon fillets, boneless
- 1 tablespoon avocado oil
- 1 red onion, sliced
- 1 teaspoon chili powder
- A pinch of salt and black pepper
- 1 teaspoon cumin, ground

Directions:
Heat up a pan with the oil over medium-high heat, add the onion and chili powder and cook for 2 minutes. Add the fish, salt, pepper and the cumin, cook for 4 minutes on each side, divide between plates and serve.

Nutrition: calories 300, fat 14, fiber 4, carbs 5, protein 20

Parsley Tuna Bowls
You just have to make these keto cakes for your family tonight!

Preparation time: 10 minutes
Cooking time: 14 minutes
Servings: 4

Ingredients:

- 1 pound tuna fillets, boneless, skinless and cubed
- 1 tablespoon olive oil
- 1 tablespoon parsley, chopped
- 2 scallions, chopped
- 1 tablespoon lime juice
- 1 teaspoon garlic powder
- A pinch of salt and black pepper

Directions:
Heat up a pan the oil over medium high heat, add the scallions and sauté for 2 minutes. Add the fish and the other ingredients, toss gently, cook for 12 more minutes, divide into bowls and serve.

Nutrition: calories 447, fat 38.7, fiber 10.3, carbs 1.1, protein 24.1

Chili Cod

Today, we recommend you to try a keto cod dish!

Preparation time: 10 minutes
Cooking time: 12 minutes
Servings: 4
Ingredients:

- 4 cod fillets, boneless
- 2 tablespoons avocado oil
- A pinch of salt and black pepper
- 1 teaspoon chili powder
- 1 tablespoon cilantro, chopped
- 3 garlic cloves, minced
- ½ teaspoon chili pepper, crushed

Directions:

Heat up a pan with the oil over medium high heat, add the garlic, chili pepper and chili powder, stir and cook for 2 minutes. Add the fish and the other ingredients, cook for 5 minutes on each side, divide between plates and serve.

Nutrition: calories 154, fat 3, fiber 0.5, carbs 4, protein 24

Baked Cod and Tomato Capers Mix

It's a very tasty and easy dish to make at home!

Preparation time: 10 minutes
Cooking time: 25 minutes
Servings: 4
Ingredients:

- 4 cod fillets, boneless
- 2 tablespoons avocado oil
- 1 cup tomato passata
- 2 tablespoons capers, drained
- 2 tablespoons parsley, chopped
- A pinch of salt and black pepper

Directions:

In a roasting pan, combine the cod with the oil and the other ingredients, toss gently, introduce in the oven at 370 degrees F and bake for 25 minutes. Divide between plates and serve.

Nutrition: calories 150, fat 3, fiber 2, carbs 0.7, protein 5

Cod and Spinach

It's an excellent keto meal!

Preparation time: 10 minutes
Cooking time: 22 minutes
Servings: 4
Ingredients:

- 4 cod fillets, boneless
- 2 shallots, chopped
- 1 cup tomato passata
- 1 tablespoon olive oil
- A pinch of salt and black pepper
- Juice of 1 lime
- 2 cups baby spinach

Directions:

Heat up a pan with the oil over medium heat, add the shallots and sauté for 2 minutes. Add the fish and cook it for 5 minutes on each side. Add the rest of the ingredients, toss gently, cook over medium heat for 10 minutes more, divide between plates and serve.

Nutrition: calories 240, fat 7.5, fiber 3, carbs 5.3, protein 10

Cod and Peppers
You are going to love this great keto idea!

Preparation time: 10 minutes
Cooking time: 18 minutes
Servings: 4

Ingredients:

- 1 red bell pepper, cut into strips
- 1 yellow bell pepper, cut into strips
- 1 green bell pepper, cut into strips
- 2 tablespoons olive oil
- 2 spring onions, chopped
- 2 garlic cloves, minced
- 4 cod fillets, boneless
- A pinch of salt and black pepper

Directions:

Heat up a pan with the oil over medium heat, add the spring onions and the garlic and sauté for 2 minutes. Add the bell peppers, toss and cook for 6 minutes more. Add the fish, salt and pepper, cook for 5 minutes on each side, divide everything between plates and serve.

Nutrition: calories 230, fat 12, fiber 1, carbs 4, protein 9

Coconut Salmon Curry
Have you ever tried a Ketogenic curry?

Preparation time: 10 minutes
Cooking time: 30 minutes
Servings: 4

Ingredients:

- 1 pound salmon fillets, boneless, skinless, cubed
- 2 tablespoons coconut oil, melted
- 2 shallots, chopped
- A pinch of salt and black pepper
- 1 teaspoon ginger powder
- 1 teaspoon curry powder
- 1 teaspoon turmeric powder
- 2 cups coconut cream
- 2 garlic cloves, minced
- ¼ cup cilantro, chopped

Directions:

Heat up a pot with the oil over medium heat, add the shallots and the garlic and sauté for 2 minutes. Add the fish, ginger, curry and turmeric powder, stir and cook for 5 minutes more. Add the remaining ingredients, bring to a simmer and cook over medium heat for 20 minutes. Divide the mix into bowls and serve.

Nutrition: calories 500, fat 34, fiber 4.1, carbs 6, protein 14.5

Shrimp and Asparagus
It's an easy and tasty idea for dinner!

Preparation time: 5 minutes
Cooking time: 10 minutes
Servings: 4

Ingredients:
- 2 tablespoons avocado oil
- 1 bunch asparagus, trimmed and halved
- 1 cup chicken stock
- 2 shallots, chopped
- 2 garlic cloves, minced
- 1 pound shrimp, peeled and deveined
- 2 tablespoons lime juice
- A pinch of salt and black pepper
- 1 tablespoon cilantro, chopped

Directions:
Heat up a pan with the oil over medium high heat, add the shallots and the garlic and sauté for 1-2 minutes. Add the shrimp, asparagus and the other ingredients, bring to a simmer and cook over medium heat for 8 minutes more. Divide everything between plates and serve.

Nutrition: calories 149, fat 1, fiber 3, carbs 1, protein 6

Sea Bass and Green Beans
This is an exceptional dish!

Preparation time: 10 minutes
Cooking time: 14 minutes
Servings: 4

Ingredients:
- 4 sea bass fillets, boneless
- 2 tablespoons olive oil
- 2 teaspoons sweet paprika
- ½ pound green beans, trimmed and halved
- 1 tablespoon lime juice
- ½ cup chicken stock
- A pinch of salt and black pepper
- 2 tablespoons parsley, chopped

Directions:
Heat up a pan with the oil over medium heat, add the fish and cook it for 2 minutes on each side. Add the green beans and the other ingredients, toss gently, bring to a simmer and cook over medium heat for 10 minutes more. Divide everything into bowls and serve.

Nutrition: calories 150, fat 4, fiber 2, carbs 1, protein 10

Shrimp and Green Onions Mix

You need to try this simple, colored and very tasty dish!

Preparation time: 10 minutes
Cooking time: 12 minutes
Servings: 4

Ingredients:

- 1 pound shrimp, peeled and deveined
- 1 tablespoon olive oil
- 4 green onions, chopped
- ½ cup cilantro, chopped
- 1 tablespoon garlic, minced
- ½ teaspoon red pepper flakes
- 1 tablespoon chives, chopped

Directions:

Heat up a pan with the oil over medium high heat, add the green onions, garlic and the pepper flakes, stir and sauté for 2 minutes. Add the shrimp and the other ingredients, bring to a simmer and cook everything for 10 minutes more. Divide the mix into bowls and serve,

Nutrition: calories 150, fat 3, fiber 3, carbs 1, protein 7

Shrimp and Avocado Mix

This keto shrimp dish is so tasty!

Preparation time: 10 minutes
Cooking time: 7 minutes
Servings: 4

Ingredients:

- 1 pound shrimp, peeled and deveined
- 1 tablespoon avocado oil
- ½ cup basil, chopped
- A pinch of salt and black pepper
- 1 avocado, peeled, pitted and cubed
- 2 tablespoons lime juice
- 2 tablespoons parsley, chopped

Directions:

Heat up a pan with the oil over medium heat, add the shrimp and cook for 4 minutes. Add the rest of the ingredients, cook over medium heat for 3 minutes more, divide into bowls and serve.

Nutrition: calories 130, fat 2, fiber 3, carbs 1, protein 6

Trout and Endives

Today, you get to try an amazing keto dish!

Preparation time: 10 minutes
Cooking time: 15 minutes
Servings: 2

Ingredients:

- 4 trout fillets
- 2 endives, shredded
- ½ cup shallots, chopped
- 2 tablespoons olive oil
- 1 teaspoon rosemary, dried
- ¼ cup chicken stock
- A pinch of salt and black pepper
- 2 tablespoons chives, chopped

Directions:

Heat up a pan with the oil over medium heat, add the shallots and the endives, toss and cook for 2 minutes. Add the fish and cook it for 2 minutes on each side. Add the rest of the ingredients, cook for 8-9 minutes more, divide between plates and serve.

Nutrition: calories 200, fat 5, fiber 2, carbs 2, protein 7

Shrimp and Fennel

You should consider making this for dinner tonight!

Preparation time: 5 minutes
Cooking time: 10 minutes
Servings: 4

Ingredients:

- 1 pound big shrimp, peeled and deveined
- 1 fennel bulb, sliced
- ¼ cup chicken stock
- 2 tablespoons olive oil
- Juice of 1 lime
- A pinch of salt and black pepper
- 1 teaspoon sweet paprika
- 1 teaspoon allspice
- 1 tablespoon cilantro, chopped

Directions:

Heat up a pan with the oil over medium heat, add the fennel and cook it for 3 minutes. Add the shrimp and the other ingredients, cook over medium heat for 7 minutes more, divide into bowls and serve.

Nutrition: calories 120, fat 3, fiber 1, carbs 2, protein 6

Shrimp and Salmon Pan

Have you ever tried something like this?

Preparation time: 10 minutes
Cooking time: 15 minutes
Servings: 4

Ingredients:

- 2 tablespoons avocado oil
- 3 shallots, minced
- 1 garlic clove, minced
- 1 pound shrimp, peeled and deveined
- ½ pound salmon fillets, boneless, skinless and cubed
- ½ cup tomato passata
- ¼ cup cilantro, chopped
- A pinch of salt and black pepper

Directions:

Heat up a pan with the oil over medium heat, add the shallots and the garlic and sauté for 2 minutes. Add the salmon and cook for 3 minutes more. Add the shrimp and the other ingredients, cook over medium heat for 10 minutes more, divide into bowls and serve.

Nutrition: calories 250, fat 12, fiber 3, carbs 5, protein 20

Shrimp and Mushroom Mix

It looks unbelievable!

Preparation time: 10 minutes
Cooking time: 15 minutes
Servings: 4

Ingredients:

- ½ pound baby bell mushrooms, sliced
- 1 pound shrimp, peeled and deveined
- 2 tablespoons olive oil
- A pinch of salt and black pepper
- 1 teaspoon red pepper flakes, crushed
- 2 garlic cloves, minced
- 1 cup heavy cream

Directions:

Heat up a pan with the oil over medium heat, add the garlic and the pepper flakes and cook for 2 minutes Add the mushrooms, toss and cook for 5 minutes more. Add the shrimp and the other ingredients, toss, cook over medium heat for 8 minutes more, divide into bowls and serve.

Nutrition: calories 455, fat 6, fiber 5, carbs 4, protein 13

Shrimp and Ginger Mix

It's one of the best ways to enjoy some shrimp!

Preparation time: 10 minutes
Cooking time: 10 minutes
Servings: 4

Ingredients:

- 2 spring onions, chopped
- 2 tablespoons coconut oil, melted
- 1 tablespoon ginger, grated
- 2 tablespoons coconut aminos
- 1 pound shrimp, peeled and deveined
- A pinch of salt and black pepper
- ½ tablespoon chives, chopped

Directions:

Heat up a pot with the oil over medium heat, add the spring onions and the ginger and cook for 2 minutes. Add the shrimp and the other ingredients, toss, cook for 8 minutes more, divide into bowls and serve.

Nutrition: calories 200, fat 3, fiber 2, carbs 4, protein 14

Calamari and Ghee Mix

You only need some simple ingredients to make this!

Preparation time: 5 minutes
Cooking time: 20 minutes
Servings: 4

Ingredients:

- 1 pound calamari rings
- ½ cup chicken stock
- 2 garlic cloves, minced
- 2 tablespoons ghee, melted
- 2 tablespoons lime juice
- 1 tablespoon parsley, chopped

Directions:

Heat up a pan with the ghee over medium heat, add the garlic and cook for 1 minute. Add the calamari and the other ingredients, toss, cook over medium heat for 18 minutes more, divide into bowls and serve.

Nutrition: calories 50, fat 1, fiber 0, carbs 0.5, protein 2

Basil Tuna
This is one of our favorite keto dishes!

Preparation time: 10 minutes
Cooking time: 14 minutes
Servings: 4

Ingredients:
- 4 tuna fillets, boneless
- 2 tablespoons olive oil
- 1 tablespoon basil, chopped
- 2 spring onions, chopped
- A pinch of salt and black pepper
- A pinch of cayenne pepper
- 1 tablespoons garlic, minced

Directions:
Heat up a pan with the oil medium heat, add the spring onions and the garlic and cook for 2 minutes more. Add the tuna and the other ingredients, cook the fish for 5 minutes on each side, divide between plates and serve.

Nutrition: calories 345, fat 32, fiber 3, carbs 3, protein 13

Baked Calamari And Shrimp
This Ketogenic seafood dish is great!

Preparation time: 10 minutes
Cooking time: 20 minutes
Servings: 1

Ingredients:
- 8 ounces calamari, cut in medium rings
- 7 ounces shrimp, peeled and deveined
- 1 eggs
- 3 tablespoons coconut flour
- 1 tablespoon coconut oil
- 2 tablespoons avocado, chopped
- 1 teaspoon tomato paste
- 1 tablespoon mayonnaise
- A splash of Worcestershire sauce
- 1 teaspoon lemon juice
- 2 lemon slices
- Salt and black pepper to the taste
- ½ teaspoon turmeric

Directions:
In a bowl, whisk egg with coconut oil. Add calamari rings and shrimp and toss to coat. In another bowl, mix flour with salt, pepper and turmeric and stir. Dredge calamari and shrimp in this mix, place everything on a lined baking sheet, introduce in the oven at 400 degrees F and bake for 10 minutes. Flip calamari and shrimp and bake for 10 minutes more. Meanwhile, in a bowl, mix avocado with mayo and tomato paste and mash using a fork. Add Worcestershire sauce, lemon juice, salt and pepper and stir well. Divide baked calamari and shrimp on plates and serve with the sauce and lemon juice on the side.

Nutrition: calories 368, fat 23, fiber 3, carbs 10, protein 34

Octopus Salad
It's so fresh and light!

Preparation time: 10 minutes
Cooking time: 40 minutes
Servings: 2

Ingredients:

- 21 ounces octopus, rinsed
- Juice from 1 lemon
- 4 celery stalks, chopped
- 3 ounces olive oil
- Salt and black pepper to the taste
- 4 tablespoons parsley, chopped

Directions:

Put the octopus in a pot, add water to cover, cover pot, bring to a boil over medium heat, cook for 40 minutes, drain and leave aside to cool down. Chop octopus and put it in a salad bowl. Add celery stalks, parsley, oil and lemon juice and toss well. Season with salt and pepper, toss again and serve.

Nutrition: calories 140, fat 10, fiber 3, carbs 6, protein 23

Clam Chowder
It's perfect for a very cold winter day!

Preparation time: 10 minutes
Cooking time: 2 hours
Servings: 4

Ingredients:

- 1 cup celery stalks, chopped
- Salt and black pepper to the taste
- 1 teaspoon thyme, ground
- 2 cups chicken stock
- 14 ounces canned baby clams
- 2 cups whipping cream
- 1 cup onion, chopped
- 13 bacon slices, chopped

Directions:

Heat up a pan over medium heat, add bacon slices, brown them and transfer to a bowl. Heat up the same pan over medium heat, add celery and onion, stir and cook for 5 minutes. Transfer everything to your Crockpot, also add bacon, baby clams, salt, pepper, stock, thyme and whipping cream, stir and cook on High for 2 hours. Divide into bowls and serve.

Nutrition: calories 420, fat 22, fiber 0, carbs 5, protein 25

Delicious Flounder And Shrimp

You just got the opportunity to learn an amazing keto recipe!

Preparation time: 10 minutes
Cooking time: 20 minutes
Servings: 4

Ingredients:

For the seasoning:

- 2 teaspoons onion powder
- 2 teaspoons thyme, dried
- 2 teaspoons sweet paprika
- 2 teaspoons garlic powder
- Salt and black pepper to the taste
- ½ teaspoon allspice, ground
- 1 teaspoon oregano, dried
- A pinch of cayenne pepper
- ¼ teaspoon nutmeg, ground
- ¼ teaspoon cloves
- A pinch of cinnamon powder

For the etouffee:

- 2 shallots, chopped
- 1 tablespoon ghee
- 8 ounces bacon, sliced

- 1 green bell pepper, chopped
- 1 celery stack, chopped
- 2 tablespoons coconut flour
- 1 tomato, chopped
- 4 garlic cloves, minced
- 8 ounces shrimp, peeled, deveined and chopped
- 2 cups chicken stock
- 1 tablespoon coconut milk
- A handful parsley, chopped
- 1 teaspoon Tabasco sauce
- Salt and black pepper to the taste

For the flounder:

- 4 flounder fillets
- 2 tablespoons ghee

Directions:

In a bowl, mix paprika with thyme, garlic and onion powder, salt, pepper, oregano, llspice, cayenne pepper, cloves, nutmeg and cinnamon and stir. Reserve 2 tablespoons of this mix, rub the flounder with the rest and leave aside. Heat up a pan over medium heat, add bacon, stir and cook for 6 minutes.Add celery, bell pepper, shallots and 1 tablespoon ghee, stir and cook for 4 minutes. Add tomato and garlic, stir and cook for 4 minutes. Add coconut flour and reserved seasoning, stir and cook for 2 minutes more. Add chicken stock and bring to a simmer. Meanwhile, heat up a pan with 2 tablespoons ghee over medium high heat, add fish, cook for 2 minutes, flip and cut for 2 minutes more. Add shrimp to the pan with the stock, stir and cook for 2 minutes. Add parsley, salt, pepper, coconut milk and Tabasco sauce, stir and take off heat. Divide fish on plates, top with the shrimp sauce and serve.

Nutrition: calories 200, fat 5, fiber 7, carbs 4, protein 20

Shrimp Salad

Serve this fresh salad tonight for dinner!

Preparation time: 10 minutes
Cooking time: 10 minutes
Servings: 4

Ingredients:

- 2 tablespoons olive oil
- 1 pound shrimp, peeled and deveined
- Salt and black pepper to the taste
- 2 tablespoons lime juice
- 3 endives, leaves separated
- 3 tablespoons parsley, chopped
- 2 teaspoons mint, chopped
- 1 tablespoon tarragon, chopped
- 1 tablespoon lemon juice
- 2 tablespoons mayonnaise
- 1 teaspoon lime zest
- ½ cup sour cream

Directions:

In a bowl, mix shrimp with salt, pepper and the olive oil, toss to coat and spread them on a lined baking sheet. Introduce shrimp in the oven at 400 degrees F and bake for 10 minutes. Add lime juice, toss them to coat again and leave aside for now. In a bowl, mix mayo with sour cream, lime zest, lemon juice, salt, pepper, tarragon, mint and parsley and stir very well. Chop shrimp, add to salad dressing, toss to coat everything and spoon into endive leaves. Serve right away.

Nutrition: calories 200, fat 11, fiber 2, carbs 1, protein 13

Delicious Oysters

This special and flavored dish is here to impress you!

Preparation time: 10 minutes
Cooking time: 0 minutes
Servings: 4

Ingredients:

- 12 oysters, shucked
- Juice from 1 lemon
- Juice from 1 orange
- Zest from 1 orange
- Juice from 1 lime
- Zest from 1 lime
- 2 tablespoons ketchup
- 1 Serrano chili pepper, chopped
- 1 cup tomato juice
- ½ teaspoon ginger, grated
- ¼ teaspoon garlic, minced
- Salt to the taste
- ¼ cup olive oil
- ¼ cup cilantro, chopped
- ¼ cup scallions, chopped

Directions:

In a bowl, mix lemon juice, orange juice, orange zest, lime juice and zest, ketchup, chili pepper, tomato juice, ginger, garlic, oil, scallions, cilantro and salt and stir well. Spoon this into oysters and serve them.

Nutrition: calories 100, fat 1, fiber 0, carbs 2, protein 5

Incredible Salmon Rolls

This Asian dish is just delicious!

Preparation time: 10 minutes
Cooking time: 0 minutes
Servings: 12

Ingredients:

- 2 nori seeds
- 1 small avocado, pitted, peeled and finely chopped
- 6 ounces smoked salmon. Sliced
- 4 ounces cream cheese
- 1 cucumber, sliced
- 1 teaspoon wasabi paste
- Picked ginger for serving

Directions:

Place nori sheets on a sushi mat. Divide salmon slices on them and also avocado and cucumber slices. In a bowl, mix cream cheese with wasabi paste and stir well. Spread this over cucumber slices, roll your nori sheets, press well, cut each in 6 pieces and serve with pickled ginger.

Nutrition: calories 80, fat 6, fiber 1, carbs 2, protein 4

Salmon Skewers

These are easy to make and they are very healthy!

Preparation time: 10 minutes
Cooking time: 8 minutes
Servings: 4

Ingredients:

- 12 ounces salmon fillet, cubed
- 1 red onion, cut in chunks
- ½ red bell pepper cut in chunks
- ½ green bell pepper cut in chunks
- ½ orange bell pepper cut in chunks
- Juice form 1 lemon
- Salt and black pepper to the taste
- A drizzle of olive oil

Directions:

Thread skewers with onion, red, green and orange pepper and salmon cubes. Season them with salt and pepper, drizzle oil and lemon juice and place them on preheated grill over medium high heat. Cook for 4 minutes on each side, divide on plates and serve.

Nutrition: calories 150, fat 3, fiber 6, carbs 3, protein 8

Grilled Shrimp
This is perfect! Just check it out!

Preparation time: 20 minutes
Cooking time: 10 minutes
Servings: 4

Ingredients:

- 1 pound shrimp, peeled and deveined
- 1 tablespoon lemon juice
- 1 garlic clove, minced
- ½ cup basil leaves
- 1 tablespoon pine nuts, toasted
- 2 tablespoons parmesan, grated
- 2 tablespoons olive oil
- Salt and black pepper to the taste

Directions:

In your food processor, mix parmesan with basil, garlic, pine nuts, oil, salt, pepper and lemon juice and blend well. Transfer this to a bowl, add shrimp, toss to coat and leave aside for 20 minutes. Thread skewers with marinated shrimp, place them on preheated grill over medium high heat, cook for 3 minutes, flip and cook for 3 more minutes. Arrange on plates and serve.

Nutrition: calories 185, fat 11, fiber 0, carbs 2, protein 13

Calamari Salad
It's an excellent choice for a summer day!

Preparation time: 30 minutes
Cooking time: 4 minutes
Servings: 4

Ingredients:

- 2 long red chilies, chopped
- 2 small red chilies, chopped
- 2 garlic cloves, minced
- 3 green onions, chopped
- 1 tablespoon balsamic vinegar
- Salt and black pepper to the taste
- Juice from 1 lemon
- 6 pounds calamari hoods, tentacles reserved
- 3.5 ounces olive oil
- 3 ounces rocket for serving

Directions:

In a bowl, mix long red chilies with small red chilies, green onions, vinegar, half of the oil, garlic, salt, pepper and lemon juice and stir well. Place calamari and tentacles in a bowl, season with salt and pepper, drizzle the rest of the oil, toss to coat and place on preheated grill over medium high heat. Cook for 2 minuets on each side and transfer to the chili marinade you've made. Toss to coat and leave aside for 30 minutes. Arrange rocket on plates, top with calamari and its marinade and serve.

Nutrition: calories 200, fat 4, fiber 2, carbs 2, protein 7

Cod Salad
It's always worth trying something new!

Preparation time: 2 hours and 10 minutes
Cooking time: 20 minutes
Servings: 8

Ingredients:

- 2 cups jarred pimiento peppers, chopped
- 2 pounds salt cod
- 1 cup parsley, chopped
- 1 cup kalamata olives, pitted and chopped
- 6 tablespoons capers
- ¾ cup olive oil
- Salt and black pepper to the taste
- Juice from 2 lemons
- 4 garlic cloves, minced
- 2 celery ribs, chopped
- ½ teaspoon red chili flakes
- 1 escarole head, leaves separated

Directions:

Put cod in a pot, add water to cover, bring to a boil over medium heat, boil for 20 minutes, drain and cut into medium chunks. Put cod in a salad bowl, add peppers, parsley, olives, capers, celery, garlic, lemon juice, salt, pepper, olive oil and chili flakes and toss to coat. Arrange escarole leaves on a platter, add cod salad and serve.

Nutrition: calories 240, fat 4, fiber 2, carbs 6, protein 9

Sardines Salad
It's a rich and nutritious winter salad you have to try soon!

Preparation time: 10 minutes
Cooking time: 0 minutes
Servings: 1

Ingredients:

- 5 ounces canned sardines in oil
- 1 tablespoons lemon juice
- 1 small cucumber, chopped
- ½ tablespoon mustard
- Salt and black pepper to the taste

Directions:

Drain sardines, put them in a bowl and mash using a fork. Add salt, pepper, cucumber, lemon juice and mustard, stir well and serve cold.

Nutrition: calories 200, fat 20, fiber 1, carbs 0, protein 20

Italian Clams Delight

It's a special Italian delight! Serve this amazing dish to your family!

Preparation time: 10 minutes
Cooking time: 10 minutes
Servings: 6

Ingredients:

- ½ cup ghee
- 36 clams, scrubbed
- 1 teaspoon red pepper flakes, crushed
- 1 teaspoon parsley, chopped
- 5 garlic cloves, minced
- 1 tablespoon oregano, dried
- 2 cups white wine

Directions:

Heat up a pan with the ghee over medium heat, add garlic, stir and cook for 1 minute. Add parsley, oregano, wine and pepper flakes and stir well. Add clams, stir, cover and cook for 10 minutes. Discard unopened clams, ladle clams and their mix into bowls and serve.

Nutrition: calories 224, fat 15, fiber 2, carbs 3, protein 4

Orange Glazed Salmon

You must try this soon! It's a delicious keto fish recipe!

Preparation time: 10 minutes
Cooking time: 10 minutes
Servings: 2

Ingredients:

- 2 lemons, sliced
- 1 pound wild salmon, skinless and cubed
- ¼ cup balsamic vinegar
- ¼ cup red orange juice
- 1 teaspoon coconut oil
- 1/3 cup orange marmalade, no sugar added

Directions:

Heat up a pot over medium heat, add vinegar, orange juice and marmalade, stir well, bring to a simmer for 1 minute, reduce temperature, cook until it thickens a bit and take off heat. Arrange salmon and lemon slices on skewers and brush them on one side with the orange glaze. Brush your kitchen grill with coconut oil and heat up over medium heat. Place salmon kebabs on grill with glazed side down and cook for 4 minutes. Flip kebabs, brush them with the rest of the orange glaze and cook for 4 minutes more. Serve right away.

Nutrition: calories 160, fat 3, fiber 2, carbs 1, protein 8

Delicious Tuna And Chimichuri Sauce

Who wouldn't love this keto dish?

Preparation time: 10 minutes
Cooking time: 5 minutes
Servings: 4
Ingredients:

- ½ cup cilantro, chopped
- 1/3 cup olive oil
- 2 tablespoons olive oil
- 1 small red onion, chopped
- 3 tablespoon balsamic vinegar
- 2 tablespoons parsley, chopped
- 2 tablespoons basil, chopped
- 1 jalapeno pepper, chopped
- 1 pound sushi grade tuna steak
- Salt and black pepper to the taste
- 1 teaspoon red pepper flakes
- 1 teaspoon thyme, chopped
- A pinch of cayenne pepper
- 3 garlic cloves, minced
- 2 avocados, pitted, peeled
- 6 ounces baby arugula

Directions:

In a bowl, mix 1/3 cup oil with jalapeno, vinegar, onion, cilantro, basil, garlic, parsley, pepper flakes, thyme, cayenne, salt and pepper, whisk well and leave aside for now. Heat up a pan with the rest of the oil over medium high heat, add tuna, season with salt and pepper, cook for 2 minutes on each side, transfer to a cutting board, leave aside to cool down a bit and slice. Mix arugula with half of the chimichuri mix you've made and toss to coat. Divide arugula on plates, top with tuna slices, drizzle the rest of the chimichuri sauce and serve with avocado slices on the side.

Nutrition: calories 186, fat 3, fiber 1, carbs 4, protein 20

Salmon Bites And Chili Sauce

This is an amazing and super tasty combination!

Preparation time: 10 minutes
Cooking time: 15 minutes
Servings: 6
Ingredients:

- 1 and ¼ cups coconut, desiccated and unsweetened
- 1 pound salmon, cubed
- 1 egg
- 1 tablespoon water
- 1/3 cup coconut flour
- 3 tablespoons coconut oil

For the sauce:

- ¼ teaspoon agar agar
- 3 garlic cloves, chopped
- ¾ cup water
- 4 Thai red chilies, chopped
- ¼ cup balsamic vinegar
- ½ cup stevia

Directions:

In a bowl, mix flour with salt and pepper and stir. In another bowl, whisk egg and 1 tablespoon water. Put the coconut in a third bowl. Dip salmon cubes in flour, egg and then in coconut and place them on a plate. Heat up a pan with the coconut oil over medium high heat, add salmon bites, cook for 3 minutes on each side and transfer them to paper towels. Heat up a pan with ¾ cup water over high heat, sprinkle agar agar and bring to a boil. Cook for 3 minutes and take off heat. In your blender, mix garlic with chilies, vinegar, stevia and a pinch of salt and blend well. Transfer this to a small pan and heat up over medium high heat. Stir, add agar mix and cook for 3 minutes.

Nutrition: calories 50, fat 2, fiber 0, carbs 4, protein 2

Irish Clams

It's an excellent idea for your dinner!

Preparation time: 10 minutes
Cooking time: 10 minutes
Servings: 4

Ingredients:

- 2 pounds clams, scrubbed
- 3 ounces pancetta
- 1 tablespoon olive oil
- 3 tablespoons ghee
- 2 garlic cloves, minced
- 1 bottle infused cider
- Salt and black pepper to the taste
- Juice from ½ lemon
- 1 small green apple, chopped
- 2 thyme springs, chopped

Directions:

Heat up a pan with the oil over medium high heat, add pancetta, brown for 3 minutes and reduce temperature to medium. Add ghee, garlic, salt, pepper and shallot, stir and cook for 3 minutes. Increase heat again, add cider, stir well and cook for 1 minute. Add clams and thyme, cover pan and simmer for 5 minutes. Discard unopened clams, add lemon juice and apple pieces, stir and divide into bowls.Serve hot.

Nutrition: calories 100, fat 2, fiber 1, carbs 1, protein 20

Seared Scallops And Roasted Grapes

A special occasion requires a special dish! Try these keto scallops!

Preparation time: 5 minutes
Cooking time: 10 minutes
Servings: 4

Ingredients:

- 1 pound scallops
- 3 tablespoons olive oil
- 1 shallot, chopped
- 3 garlic cloves, minced
- 2 cups spinach
- 1 cup chicken stock
- 1 romanesco lettuce head
- 1 and ½ cups red grapes, cut in halves
- ¼ cup walnuts, toasted and chopped
- 1 tablespoon ghee
- Salt and black pepper to the taste

Directions:

Put romanesco in your food processor, blend and transfer to a bowl. Heat up a pan with 2 tablespoons oil over medium high heat, add shallot and garlic, stir and cook for 1 minute. Add romanesco, spinach and 1 cup stock, stir, cook for 3 minutes, blend using an immersion blender and take off heat. Heat up another pan with 1 tablespoon oil and the ghee over medium high heat, add scallops, season with salt and pepper, cook for 2 minutes, flip and sear for 1 minute more. Divide romanesco mix on plates, add scallops on the side, top with walnuts and grapes and serve.

Nutrition: calories 300, fat 12, fiber 2, carbs 6, protein 20

Oysters And Pico De Gallo

It's flavored and very delicious!

Preparation time: 10 minutes
Cooking time: 10 minutes
Servings: 6
Ingredients:

- 18 oysters, scrubbed
- A handful cilantro, chopped
- 2 tomatoes, chopped
- 1 jalapeno pepper, chopped
- ¼ cup red onion, finely chopped
- Salt and black pepper to the taste
- ½ cup Monterey Jack cheese, shredded
- 2 limes, cut in wedges
- Juice from 1 lime

Directions:

In a bowl, mix onion with jalapeno, cilantro, tomatoes, salt, pepper and lime juice and stir well. Place oysters on preheated grill over medium high heat, cover grill and cook for 7 minutes until they open. Transfer opened oysters to a heat proof dish and discard unopened ones. Top oysters with cheese and introduce in preheated broiler for 1 minute. Arrange oysters on a platter, top each with tomatoes mix you've made earlier and serve with lime wedges on the side.

Nutrition: calories 70, fat 2, fiber 0, carbs 1, protein 1

Grilled Squid And Tasty Guacamole

The squid combines perfectly with the delicious guacamole!

Preparation time: 10 minutes
Cooking time: 10 minutes
Servings: 2
Ingredients:

- 2 medium squids, tentacles separated and tubes scored lengthwise
- A drizzle of olive oil
- Juice from 1 lime
- Salt and black pepper to the taste

For the guacamole:

- 2 avocados, pitted, peeled and chopped
- Some coriander springs, chopped
- 2 red chilies, chopped
- 1 tomato, chopped
- 1 red onion, chopped
- Juice from 2 limes

Directions:

Season squid and squid tentacles with salt, pepper, drizzle some olive oil and massage well. Place on preheated grill over medium high heat score side down and cook for 2 minutes. Flip and cook for 2 minutes more and transfer to a bowl. Add juice from 1 lime, toss to coat and keep warm. Put avocado in a bowl and mash using a fork. Add coriander, chilies, tomato, onion and juice from 2 limes and stir well everything. Divide squid on plates, top with guacamole and serve.

Nutrition: calories 500, fat 43, fiber 6, carbs 7, protein 20

Shrimp And Cauliflower Delight

It's look good and it tastes amazing!

Preparation time: 10 minutes
Cooking time: 15 minutes
Servings: 2
Ingredients:

- 1 tablespoon ghee
- 1 cauliflower head
- 1 pound shrimp
- ¼ cup coconut milk
- 8 ounces mushrooms chopped
- 2 garlic cloves, minced
- 4 bacon slices
- ½ cup beef stock
- 1 tablespoon parsley,
- 1 tablespoon chives, chopped

Directions:

Heat up a pan over medium high heat, add bacon, cook until it's crispy, transfer to paper towels and leave aside. Heat up another pan with 1 tablespoon bacon fat over medium high heat, add shrimp, cook for 2 minutes on each side and transfer to a bowl. Heat up the pan again over medium heat, add mushrooms, stir and cook for 3-4 minutes. Add garlic, pepper flakes, stir and cook for 1 minute. Add beef stock, salt, pepper and return shrimp to pan as well. Stir, cook until everything thickens a bit, take off heat and keep warm. Meanwhile, put cauliflower in your food processor and mince it. Place this into a heated pan over medium high heat, stir and cook fro 5 minutes. Add ghee and butter, stir and blend using an immersion blender. Add salt and pepper to the taste, stir and divide into bowls. Top with shrimp mix and serve with parsley and chives sprinkled all over.

Nutrition: calories 245, fat 7, fiber 4, carbs 6, protein 20

Salmon Stuffed With Shrimp

It will soon become one of your favorite keto recipes!

Preparation time: 10 minutes
Cooking time: 25 minutes
Servings: 2
Ingredients:

- 2 salmon fillets
- A drizzle of olive oil
- 5 ounces tiger shrimp,
- 6 mushrooms, chopped
- 3 green onions, chopped
- 2 cups spinach
- ¼ cup macadamia nuts, toasted
- A pinch of nutmeg
- ¼ cup mayonnaise

Directions:

Heat up a pan with the oil over medium high heat, add mushrooms, onions, salt and pepper, stir and cook for 4 minutes. Add macadamia nuts, stir and cook for 2 minutes. Add spinach, stir and cook for 1 minute. Add shrimp, stir and cook for 1 minutes. Take off heat, leave aside for a few minutes, add mayo and nutmeg and stir well. Make an incision lengthwise in each salmon fillet, sprinkle salt and pepper, divide spinach and shrimp mix into incisions and place on a working surface. Heat up a pan with a drizzle of oil over medium high heat, add stuffed salmon, skin side down, cook for 1 minutes, reduce temperature, cover pan and cook for 8 minutes. Broil for 3 minutes, divide on plates and serve.

Nutrition: calories 430, fat 30, fiber 3, carbs 7, protein 50

Mustard Glazed Salmon

This is one of our favorite keto salmon dish! You will feel the same!

Preparation time: 10 minutes
Cooking time: 20 minutes
Servings: 1
Ingredients:

- 1 big salmon fillet
- Salt and black pepper to the taste
- 2 tablespoons mustard
- 1 tablespoon coconut oil
- 1 tablespoon maple extract

Directions:

In a bowl, mix maple extract with mustard and whisk well. Season salmon with salt and pepper and brush salmon with half of the mustard mix Heat up a pan with the oil over medium high heat, place salmon flesh side down and cook for 5 minutes. Brush salmon with the rest of the mustard mix, transfer to a baking dish, introduce in the oven at 425 degrees F and bake for 15 minutes. Serve with a tasty side salad.

Nutrition: calories 240, fat 7, fiber 1, carbs 5, protein 23

Incredible Salmon Dish

You will make this over and over again!

Preparation time: 10 minutes
Cooking time: 15 minutes
Servings: 4
Ingredients:

- 3 cups ice water
- 2 teaspoons sriracha sauce
- 4 teaspoons stevia
- 3 scallions, chopped
- Salt and black pepper to the taste
- 2 teaspoons flaxseed oil
- 4 teaspoons apple cider vinegar
- 3 teaspoons avocado oil
- 4 medium salmon fillets
- 4 cups baby arugula
- 2 cups cabbage, finely chopped
- 1 and ½ teaspoon Jamaican jerk seasoning
- ¼ cup pepitas, toasted
- 2 cups watermelon radish, julienned

Directions:

Put ice water in a bowl, add scallions and leave aside. In another bowl, mix sriracha sauce with stevia and stir well. Transfer 2 teaspoons of this mix to a bowl and mix with half of the avocado oil, flaxseed oil, vinegar, salt and pepper and whisk well. Sprinkle jerk seasoning over salmon, rub with sriracha and stevia mix and season with salt and pepper. Heat up a pan with the rest of the avocado oil over medium high heat, add salmon, flesh side down, cook for 4 minutes, flip and cook for 4 minutes more and divide on plates. In a bowl, mix radishes with cabbage and arugula. Add salt, pepper, sriracha and vinegar mix and toss well. Add this next to salmon fillets, drizzle the remaining sriracha and stevia sauce all over and top with pepitas and drained scallions.

Nutrition: calories 160, fat 6, fiber 1, carbs 1, protein 12

Scallops And Fennel Sauce

It contains a lot of healthy elements and it's easy to make! Try it if you are on a keto diet!

Preparation time: 10 minutes
Cooking time: 10 minutes
Servings: 2

Ingredients:

- 6 scallops
- 1 fennel, trimmed, leaves chopped and bulbs cut in wedges
- Juice from ½ lime
- 1 lime, cut in wedges
- Zest from 1 lime
- 1 egg yolk
- 3 tablespoons ghee, melted and heated up
- ½ tablespoons olive oil

Directions:

Season scallops with salt and pepper, put in a bowl and mix with half of the lime juice and half of the zest and toss to coat. In a bowl, mix egg yolk with some salt and pepper, the rest of the lime juice and the rest of the lime zest and whisk well. Add melted ghee and stir very well. Also add fennel leaves and stir. Brush fennel wedges with oil, place on heated grill over medium high heat, cook for 2 minutes, flip and cook for 2 minutes more. Add scallops on grill, cook for 2 minutes, flip and cook for 2 minutes more. Divide fennel and scallops on plates, drizzle fennel and ghee mix and serve with lime wedges on the side.

Nutrition: calories 400, fat 24, fiber 4, carbs 12, protein 25

Salmon And Lemon Relish

Enjoy a slow cooked salmon and a delicious relish!

Preparation time: 10 minutes
Cooking time: 1 hour
Servings: 2

Ingredients:

- 2 medium salmon fillets
- Salt and black pepper to the taste
- A drizzle of olive oil
- 1 shallot, chopped
- 1 tablespoon lemon juice
- 1 big lemon
- ¼ cup olive oil
- 2 tablespoons parsley, finely chopped

Directions:

Brush salmon fillets with a drizzle of olive oil, sprinkle with salt and pepper, place on a lined baking sheet, introduce in the oven at 400 degrees F and bake for 1 hour. Meanwhile, put shallot in a bowl, add 1 tablespoon lemon juice, salt and pepper, stir and leave aside for 10 minutes. Cut the whole lemon in wedges and then very thinly. Add this to shallots, also add parsley and ¼ cup olive oil and stir everything. Take salmon out of the oven, break into medium pieces and serve with the lemon relish on the side.

Nutrition: calories 200, fat 10, fiber 1, carbs 5, protein 20

Mussels Soup
Oh my God! This is so good!

Preparation time: 10 minutes
Cooking time: 15 minutes
Servings: 6
Ingredients:

- 2 pounds mussels
- 28 ounces canned tomatoes, crushed
- 28 ounces canned tomatoes, chopped
- 2 cup chicken stock
- 1 teaspoon red pepper flakes, crushed
- 3 garlic cloves, minced
- 1 handful parsley, chopped
- 1 yellow onion, chopped
- 1 tablespoon olive oil

Directions:

Heat up a Dutch oven with the oil over medium high heat, add onion, stir and cook for 3 minutes. Add garlic and red pepper flakes, stir and cook for 1 minute. Add crushed and chopped tomatoes and stir. Add chicken stock, salt and pepper, stir and bring to a boil. Add rinsed mussels, salt and pepper, cook until they open, discard unopened ones and mix with parsley. Stir, divide into bowls and serve.

Nutrition: calories 250, fat 3, fiber 3, carbs 2, protein 8

Swordfish And Mango Salsa
The mango salsa is divide! Just serve it with the swordfish!

Preparation time: 10 minutes
Cooking time: 6 minutes
Servings: 2
Ingredients:

- 2 medium swordfish steaks
- Salt and black pepper to the taste
- 2 teaspoons avocado oil
- 1 tablespoon cilantro, chopped
- 1 mango, chopped
- 1 avocado, pitted, peeled and chopped
- A pinch of cumin
- A pinch of onion powder
- A pinch of garlic powder
- 1 orange, peeled and sliced
- ½ balsamic vinegar

Directions:

Season fish steaks with salt, pepper, garlic powder, onion powder and cumin. Heat up a pan with half of the oil over medium high eat, add fish steaks and cook them for 3 minutes on each side. Meanwhile, in a bowl, mix avocado with mango, cilantro, balsamic vinegar, salt, pepper and the rest of the oil and stir well. Divide fish on plates, top with mango salsa and serve with orange slices on the side.

Nutrition: calories 160, fat 3, fiber 2, carbs 4, protein 8

Tasty Sushi Bowl

It's a tasty recipe full of great ingredients!

Preparation time: 10 minutes
Cooking time: 7 minutes
Servings: 4
Ingredients:

- 1 ahi tuna steak
- 2 tablespoons coconut oil
- 1 cauliflower head
- 2 tablespoons green onions,
- 1 avocado, pitted, peeled and
- 1 cucumber, grated
- 1 nori sheet, torn
- Some cloves sprouts

For the salad dressing:

- 1 tablespoon sesame oil
- 2 tablespoons coconut aminos
- 1 tablespoon apple cider vinegar
- 1 teaspoon stevia

Directions:

Put cauliflower florets in your food processor and blend until you obtain a cauliflower "rice". Put some water in a pot, add a steamer basket inside, add cauliflower rice, bring to a boil over medium heat, cover, steam for a few minutes, drain and transfer "rice" to a bowl. Heat up a pan with the coconut oil over medium high heat, add tuna, cook for 1 minute on each side and transfer to a cutting board. Divide cauliflower rice into bowls, top with nori pieces, cloves sprouts, cucumber, green onions and avocado. In a bowl, mix sesame oil with vinegar, coconut aminos, salt and stevia and whisk well. Drizzle this over cauliflower rice and mixed veggies, top with tuna pieces and serve.

Nutrition: calories 300, fat 12, fiber 6, carbs 6, protein 15

Tasty Grilled Swordfish

You don't need to be an expert cook to make this tasty keto dish!

Preparation time: 3 hours and 10 minutes
Cooking time: 10 minutes
Servings: 4
Ingredients:

- 1 tablespoon parsley, chopped
- 1 lemon, cut in wedges
- 4 swordfish steaks
- 3 garlic cloves, minced
- 1/3 cup chicken stock
- 3 tablespoons olive oil
- ¼ cup lemon juice
- Salt and black pepper to the taste
- ½ teaspoon rosemary, dried
- ½ teaspoon sage, dried
- ½ teaspoon marjoram, dried

Directions:

In a bowl, mix chicken stock with garlic, lemon juice, olive oil, salt, pepper, sage, marjoram and rosemary and whisk well. Add swordfish steaks, toss to coat and keep in the fridge for 3 hours. Place marinated fish steaks on preheated grill over medium high heat and cook for 5 minutes on each side. Arrange on plates, sprinkle parsley on to and serve with lemon wedges on the side.

Nutrition: calories 136, fat 5, fiber 0, carbs 1, protein 20

Ketogenic Poultry Recipes

Ghee Chicken Mix
This is perfect for a friendly meal!

Preparation time: 10 minutes
Cooking time: 20 minutes
Servings: 4

Ingredients:

- 2 tablespoons garlic powder
- 2 chicken breasts, skinless boneless and sliced
- Salt and black pepper to the taste
- ½ cup ghee, melted
- ½ cup chicken stock
- 1 tablespoon cilantro, chopped

Directions:

Heat up a pan with the ghee over medium heat, add the chicken and cook for 5 minutes on each side. Add the rest of the ingredients, cook for 10 minutes more, divide between plates and serve.

Nutrition: calories 439, fat 33.4, fiber 0.4, carbs 3.2, protein 31.3

Paprika Chicken Wings
It's so fresh and delicious!

Preparation time: 10 minutes
Cooking time: 20 minutes
Servings: 4

Ingredients:

- 1 pound chicken wings
- 1 tablespoon cumin, ground
- 1 teaspoon coriander, ground
- 1 tablespoon sweet paprika
- A pinch of salt and black pepper
- 1 tablespoon lime juice
- 2 tablespoons olive oil

Directions:

In a bowl, mix the chicken wings with the cumin and the other ingredients, toss, spread them on a baking sheet lined with parchment paper and cook at 420 degrees F for 20 minutes. Divide between plates and serve.

Nutrition: calories 286, fat 16, fiber 0.8, carbs 1.6, protein 33.3

Chicken and Capers

Hurry up and make this dish today!

Preparation time: 10 minutes
Cooking time: 15 minutes
Servings: 4

Ingredients:

- 1 pound chicken breast, skinless, boneless and sliced
- 1 tablespoon olive oil
- 1 tablespoons capers, drained
- 1 cup tomato passata
- A pinch of salt and black pepper
- 1 tablespoon parsley, chopped

Directions:

Heat up a pan with the oil over medium heat, add the chicken and cook for 4 minutes on each side. Add the rest of the ingredients, cook for 8 minutes more, divide between plates and serve.

Nutrition: calories 166, fat 6.4, fiber 0.6, carbs 1.2, protein 24.6

Cilantro Wings

You will have these done in no time!

Preparation time: 10 minutes
Cooking time: 20 minutes
Servings: 4

Ingredients:

- 2 pounds chicken wings
- Juice of 1 lime
- 1 tablespoon olive oil
- ¼ cup cilantro, chopped
- 2 garlic cloves, minced
- A pinch of salt and black pepper

Directions:

In a bowl, mix the chicken wings with the lime juice and the other ingredients, toss and transfer them to a roasting pan. Introduce in the oven and cook at 390 degrees F for 20 minutes. Divide the chicken wings between plates and serve with a side dish.

Nutrition: calories 463, fat 20.3, fiber 0.1, carbs 0.6, protein 65.7

Baked Turkey Mix
It's a very simple keto chicken recipe!

Preparation time: 10 minutes
Cooking time: 30 minutes
Servings: 4

Ingredients:

- 1 big turkey breast, skinless, boneless and sliced
- 3 green onions, chopped
- ½ cup tomato passata
- 1 tablespoon avocado oil
- 1 cup green olives, pitted and halved
- 2 tablespoons parmesan, grated

Directions:

Grease a baking dish with the oil, arrange the turkey slices inside, add the onions and the other ingredients except the parmesan and toss. Sprinkle the parmesan on top, ntroduce the dish in the oven and bake at 390 degrees F for 30 minutes. Divide the mix between plates and serve.

Nutrition: calories 450, fat 24, fiber 0, carbs 3, protein 60

Turkey and Artichokes Mix
This is an Italian style keto dish we really appreciate!

Preparation time: 10 minutes
Cooking time: 25 minutes
Servings: 4

Ingredients:

- 2 tablespoons olive oil
- 1 red onion, chopped
- 1 cup chicken stock
- 1 big turkey breast, skinless, boneless and sliced
- 2 artichokes, trimmed and quartered
- 4 garlic cloves, minced
- A pinch of salt and black pepper
- ½ teaspoon red chili flakes
- 1 tablespoon cilantro, chopped

Directions:

Heat up a pan with the oil over medium heat, add the turkey and cook for 5 minutes. Add the onion and the other ingredients, cook everything over medium heat for 20 minutes more, divide between plates and serve.

Nutrition: calories 400, fat 20, fiber 1, carbs 2, protein 7

Curry Chicken
You'll soon see how easy this keto recipe is!

Preparation time: 10 minutes
Cooking time: 30 minutes
Servings: 4

Ingredients:

- 1 pound chicken breast, skinless, boneless and cubed
- 1 tablespoon olive oil
- 1 tablespoon yellow curry paste
- 1 cup chicken stock
- A pinch of salt and black pepper
- 1 teaspoon sweet paprika
- ½ teaspoon allspice, ground
- 1 tablespoon cilantro, chopped

Directions:
Heat up a pan with the oil over medium heat, add the meat and brown it for 5 minutes. Add the curry paste and he other ingredients, toss, bring to a simmer and cook for 25 minutes Divide the mix into bowls and serve.

Nutrition: calories 334, fat 24, fiber 2, carbs 4.5, protein 27

Turkey and Coconut Sauce
It's very healthy and it will make a great dinner idea!

Preparation time: 10 minutes
Cooking time: 30 minutes
Servings: 4

Ingredients:

- 1 tablespoon coconut oil, melted
- 1 turkey breast, skinless, boneless and cubed
- 1 cup chicken stock
- 2 shallots, chopped
- ¼ cup coconut milk
- 2 tablespoons parsley, chopped
- A pinch of salt and black pepper

Directions:
Heat up a pan with the oil over medium high heat, add the shallots and the meat and brown for 5 minutes. Add the stock and the other ingredients, bring to a simmer and cook for 25 minutes stirring often. Divide into bowls and serve.

Nutrition: calories 112, fat 7.9, fiber 0.6, carbs 3, protein 7.9

Coriander Chicken Mix
Try this next idea today!

Preparation time: 10 minutes
Cooking time: 20 minutes
Servings: 4

Ingredients:

- 2 pounds chicken breasts, skinless, boneless and cubed
- 2 teaspoons cumin, ground
- 2 tablespoons avocado oil
- 2 tablespoons lime juice
- A pinch of salt and black pepper
- 1 teaspoon coriander, ground
- 1 tablespoon cilantro, chopped

Directions:

Heat up the pan with the oil over medium heat, add the chicken and brown it for 5 minutes. Add the cumin and the other ingredients, toss, cook over medium heat for 15 minutes more, divide between plates and serve with a side salad.

Nutrition: calories 240, fat 10, fiber 2, carbs 5, protein 20

Baked Tarragon Turkey
The combination is absolutely delicious! We guarantee it!

Preparation time: 10 minutes
Cooking time: 30 minutes
Servings: 4

Ingredients:

- 1 pound turkey breast, skinless, boneless and sliced
- 2 tablespoons olive oil
- 1 cup chicken stock
- A pinch of salt and black pepper
- 1 tablespoon tarragon, chopped

Directions:

In a roasting pan, combine the meat with the oil and the other ingredients, toss gently and bake at 390 degrees F for 30 minutes. Divide the turkey mix between plates and serve with a side salad.

Nutrition: calories 182, fat 9.1, fiber 0.6, carbs 5.2, protein 19.6

Chicken and Salsa
Everyone will be impressed with this keto dish!

Preparation time: 10 minutes
Cooking time: 20 minutes
Servings: 4

Ingredients:

- 2 pounds chicken breasts, skinless, boneless and cubed
- 2 tablespoons olive oil
- ½ cup chicken stock
- 2 shallots, chopped
- 1 cup cherry tomatoes, halved
- 1 cup cucumber, cubed
- 1 cup black olives, pitted and sliced
- ¼ cup parsley, chopped
- 1 tablespoons lime juice

Directions:

Heat up a pan with the oil over medium heat, add the shallots, toss and cook for 2 minutes. Add the chicken and brown for 5 minutes more. Add the tomatoes and the other ingredients, toss, cook over medium heat for 12-13 minutes more, divide into bowls and serve.

Nutrition: calories 230, fat 12, fiber 5.0, carbs 6.3, protein 20

Creamy Turkey
It's an extravagant dish but it's worth trying!

Preparation time: 10 minutes
Cooking time: 30 minutes
Servings: 4

Ingredients:

- 1 pound turkey breast, skinless, boneless and cubed
- 1 cup heavy cream
- 2 tablespoons olive oil
- 2 spring onions, chopped
- 2 leeks, chopped
- A pinch of salt and black pepper
- 1 tablespoon cilantro, chopped

Directions:

Heat up a pan with the oil over medium heat, add the spring onions and the leeks and sauté for 2 minutes. Add the meat and brown for 3 minutes more. Add the rest of the ingredients, bring to a simmer and cook over medium heat for 25 minutes more, stirring often. Divide the mix into bowls and serve.

Nutrition: calories 267, fat 5.6, fiber 0, carbs 6.0, protein 35

Duck and Zucchinis

If you are really hungry today then you should really try this recipe!

Preparation time: 10 minutes
Cooking time: 35 minutes
Servings: 4

Ingredients:

- 1 pound duck breasts, skinless, boneless and roughly cubed
- 2 zucchinis, sliced
- 1 tablespoon avocado oil
- 2 shallots, chopped
- ½ teaspoon chili powder
- 1 cup chicken stock
- A pinch of salt and black pepper

Directions:

Heat up a pan with the oil over medium high heat, add the shallots, stir and sauté for 5 minutes. Add the meat and the other ingredients, toss, bring to a simmer and cook over medium heat for 30 minutes. Divide the mix into bowls and serve.

Nutrition: calories 450, fat 23, fiber 3, carbs 8.3, protein 50

Chicken and Raspberries Salad

It's a tasty salad and so easy to make!

Preparation time: 10 minutes
Cooking time: 20 minutes
Servings: 4

Ingredients:

- 1 shallot, chopped
- 2 tablespoons olive oil
- 2 tablespoons balsamic vinegar
- ¼ cup chicken stock
- 1 cup raspberries
- 1 pound chicken breast, skinless, boneless and cut into strips
- 2 cups baby spinach
- 1 tablespoon cilantro, chopped

Directions:

Heat up a pan with the oil over medium heat, add the shallot and the chicken and brown for 5 minutes. Add the remaining ingredients, toss, cook over medium heat for 15 minutes more, divide into bowls and serve.

Nutrition: calories 245, fat 13.40, fiber 4, carbs 5.6, protein 18

Turkey and Spinach
It's a great way to end your day!

Preparation time: 10 minutes
Cooking time: 40 minutes
Servings: 6

Ingredients:

- 2 tablespoons olive oil
- 1 pound turkey breast, skinless, boneless and sliced
- 1 cup baby spinach
- 2 shallots, chopped
- A pinch of salt and black pepper
- Salt and black pepper to the taste
- ¼ teaspoon sweet paprika
- ¼ teaspoon garlic powder
- 1 tablespoon cilantro, chopped

Directions:

Heat up a pan with the oil over medium heat, add the meat and the shallots and brown for 5 minutes. Add the spinach and the other ingredients, toss, bring to a simmer and cook over medium heat for 20 minutes. Divide the mix in to bowls and serve.

Nutrition: calories 320, fat 23, fiber 8, carbs 6, protein 16

Turkey and Tomatoes
It's a very comforting and rich mix!

Preparation time: 10 minutes
Cooking time: 30 minutes
Servings: 4

Ingredients:

- 2 shallots, chopped
- 1 tablespoon ghee, melted
- 1 cup chicken stock
- 1 pound turkey breast, skinless, boneless and cubed
- 1 cup cherry tomatoes, halved
- A pinch of salt and black pepper
- 1 tablespoon rosemary, chopped

Directions:

Heat up a pan with the ghee over medium high heat, add the shallots and the meat and brown for 5 minutes. Add the rest of the ingredients, bring to a simmer and cook over medium heat for 25 minutes, stirring often. Divide into bowls and serve.

Nutrition: calories 150, fat 4, fiber 1, carbs 3, protein 10

Turkey and Cabbage Mix

Try it soon! You will make it a second time as well!

Preparation time: 10 minutes
Cooking time: 30 minutes
Servings: 4

Ingredients:

- 1 red cabbage, shredded
- 1 pound turkey breast, skinless, boneless and cubed
- 2 tablespoons olive oil
- 2 garlic cloves, mined
- 2 spring onions, chopped
- 1 cup tomato passata
- 1 tablespoon cilantro, chopped
- A pinch of salt and black pepper

Directions:

Heat up a pan with the oil over medium heat, add the onions and the garlic and sauté for 2 minutes. Add the meat and brown for 6 minutes more. Add the rest of the ingredients, toss, bring to a simmer and cook over medium heat for 20 minutes more. Divide everything into bowls and serve.

Nutrition: calories 240, fat 15, fiber 1, carbs 3, protein 25

Chili Turkey and Broccoli

This great keto dish is perfect for a cold and rainy day!

Preparation time: 10 minutes
Cooking time: 30 minutes
Servings: 4

Ingredients:

- 1 pound turkey breast, skinless, boneless and cubed
- 1 cup broccoli florets
- 1 cup chicken stock
- 2 shallots, chopped
- 1 tablespoon olive oil
- A pinch of salt and black pepper
- 1 teaspoon chili powder
- 1 tablespoon chipotle peppers, chopped
- ½ teaspoon garlic powder
- 1 tablespoon cilantro, chopped

Directions:

Heat up a pan with the oil over medium heat, add the shallots and the meat and brown for 10 minutes. Add the stock and the other ingredients except the cilantro, toss, bring to a simmer and cook over medium heat for 20 minutes more. Add the cilantro, stir, divide into bowls and serve.

Nutrition: calories 154, fat 5, fiber 3, carbs 2, protein 27

Ground Turkey and Bell Peppers
You will make this in no time!

Preparation time: 10 minutes
Cooking time: 30 minutes
Servings: 4

Ingredients:

- 1 pound turkey meat, ground
- 1 tablespoon olive oil
- 3 garlic cloves, minced
- 1 cup tomatoes, chopped
- 1 red bell pepper, cut into strips
- 1 green bell pepper, cut into strips
- A pinch of salt and black pepper
- 1 tablespoon coriander, ground
- 2 tablespoons ginger, grated
- 2 tablespoons chili powder

Directions:

Heat up a pan with the oil over medium heat, add the garlic and the meat and brown for 5 minutes. Add the bell pepper, and cook for 5 minutes more. Add the rest of the ingredients, toss, bring to a simmer and cook over medium heat for 20 minutes more. Divide everything into bowls and serve.

Nutrition: calories 240, fat 4, fiber 3, carbs 2, protein 12

Chicken and Walnuts Salad
It's healthy, it's fresh and very delicious!

Preparation time: 10 minutes
Cooking time: 0 minutes
Servings: 4

Ingredients:

- 2 cups baby arugula
- 2 cups rotisserie chicken, skinless, boneless and shredded
- 3 tablespoons walnuts, chopped
- 2 tablespoons olive oil
- 2 tablespoon lime juice
- A pinch of salt and black pepper
- 1 tablespoon chives, chopped

Directions:

In a salad bowl, combine the chicken with the walnuts, arugula and the other ingredients, toss and serve.

Nutrition: calories 120, fat 2, fiber 1, carbs 3, protein 7

Chicken and Kale Mix

This sounds really great, doesn't it?

Preparation time: 10 minutes
Cooking time: 25 minutes
Servings: 4

Ingredients:

- 1 pound chicken breast, skinless, boneless and cubed
- 2 tablespoons avocado oil
- 1 cup kale, torn
- 2 shallots, chopped
- 1 teaspoon chili powder
- ½ cup tomato passata
- A pinch of salt and black pepper
- 1 tablespoon parsley, chopped

Directions:

Heat up a pan with the oil over medium high heat, add the shallots and the chili powder, stir and cook for 5 minutes. Add the meat and brown it for 5 minutes more. Add the kale and the other ingredients, toss, cook over medium heat for 15 minutes more, divide between plates and serve.

Nutrition: calories 290, fat 12, fiber 2, carbs 4, protein 24

Mozzarella Chicken

This is a magnificent combination of ingredients!

Preparation time: 10 minutes
Cooking time: 30 minutes
Servings: 4

Ingredients:

- 1 pound chicken breast, skinless, boneless and cubed
- 1 tablespoon olive oil
- 2 shallots, chopped
- 1 cup tomatoes, cubed
- A pinch of salt and black pepper
- 1 cup mozzarella, shredded
- 1 tablespoon chives, chopped
- ¼ teaspoon sweet paprika

Directions:

Heat up a pan with the oil over medium high heat, add the shallots and sauté for 2 minutes. Add the chicken and brown for 5 minutes more. Add the other ingredients except the cheese and toss. Sprinkle the cheese on top, introduce the pan in the oven and bake at 390 degrees F for 15 minutes. Divide everything between plates and serve.

Nutrition: calories 223, fat 8, fiber 1, carbs 3, protein 26

Salsa Turkey
Try this great keto dish today!

Preparation time: 10 minutes
Cooking time: 35 minutes
Servings: 4

Ingredients:

- 1 turkey breast, skinless, boneless and sliced
- 2 tablespoons olive oil
- 1 cup chicken stock
- 1 cup salsa Verde
- A pinch of salt and black pepper

Directions:
In a baking dish, combine the meat with the oil and the other ingredients, toss, introduce in the oven at 400 degrees F and bake for 35 minutes. Divide everything between plates and serve.

Nutrition: calories 120, fat 2, fiber 2, carbs 6, protein 10

Chicken and Mushrooms
You should consider trying this Italian keto dish as soon as possible!

Preparation time: 10 minutes
Cooking time: 30 minutes
Servings: 4

Ingredients:

- 1 pound chicken breast, skinless, boneless and cubed
- 2 cups baby bella mushrooms, sliced
- 2 tablespoons olive oil
- 1 red onion, chopped
- 1 red bell pepper, chopped
- 2 garlic cloves, minced
- A pinch of salt and black pepper
- ½ cup chicken stock
- 1 tablespoon balsamic vinegar
- 1 tablespoon parsley, chopped

Directions:
Heat up a pan with the oil over medium heat, add the onion and the mushrooms, stir and cook for 5 minutes. Add the chicken, toss and brown for 5 minutes more. Add the rest of the ingredients, toss, bring to a simmer and cook over medium heat for 20 minutes. Divide everything between plates and serve.

Nutrition: calories 340, fat 33, fiber 3, carbs 4, protein 20

Chicken and Zucchini Casserole
This could be your lunch today!

Preparation time: 10 minutes
Cooking time: 40 minutes
Servings: 4

Ingredients:

- 2 pounds chicken breast, skinless and boneless and sliced
- 2 tablespoons olive oil
- 2 spring onions, chopped
- 2 zucchinis, roughly cubed
- A pinch of salt and black pepper
- 1 teaspoon oregano, dried
- 1 teaspoon basil, dried
- 1 cup tomato passata
- 1 cup parmesan, grated
- 1 tablespoon parsley, chopped

Directions:

Heat up a pan with the oil over medium high heat, add the spring onions and sauté for 2 minutes. Add the chicken and cook for 2 minutes on each side. Transfer this to a baking dish, add the zucchinis and the other ingredients except the cheese and the parsley. Sprinkle the cheese and the parsley on top, introduce the oven and bake at 375 degrees F for 35 minutes. Divide the mix between plates and serve.

Nutrition: calories 300, fat 6, fiber 3, carbs 5, protein 28

Chicken and Cauliflower
These will really impress your guests!

Preparation time: 10 minutes
Cooking time: 30 minutes
Servings: 4

Ingredients:

- 2 cups cauliflower florets
- 1 pound chicken breast, skinless, boneless and cubed
- 2 tablespoons olive oil
- 2 shallots, chopped
- A pinch of salt and black pepper
- 1 cup chicken stock
- 1 teaspoon sweet paprika
- 1 cup mozzarella, shredded

Directions:

Heat up a pan with the oil over medium heat, add the shallots and sauté for 5 minutes. Add the chicken and brown for 5 minutes more. Add the rest of the ingredients except the cheese and toss gently. Sprinkle the cheese on top, introduce in the oven at 350 degrees F and bake for 20 minutes. Divide everything between plates and serve.

Nutrition: calories 200, fat 6, fiber 3, carbs 6, protein 14

Chicken and Garlic Green Beans
This is a really delicious keto chicken dish!

Preparation time: 10 minutes
Cooking time: 30 minutes
Servings: 4

Ingredients:
- 1 pound chicken breast, skinless and boneless and roughly cubed
- 2 tablespoons avocado oil
- 2 shallots, chopped
- ½ pound green beans, trimmed and halved
- 4 garlic cloves, mined
- 1 cup chicken stock
- ½ cup tomato passata
- 1 tablespoon cilantro, chopped
- A pinch of salt and black pepper

Directions:
Heat up a pan with the oil over medium heat, add the shallots and the meat and brown for 5 minutes. Add the garlic and the green beans, and cook for 5 minutes more. Add the rest of the ingredients, toss gently, bring to a simmer and cook over medium heat for 20 minutes more. Divide between plates and serve.

Nutrition: calories 240, fat 4, fiber 3, carbs 6, protein 20

Chicken and Broccoli Casserole
You must really make this tonight!

Preparation time: 10 minutes
Cooking time: 35 minutes
Servings: 4

Ingredients:
- 1 pound chicken breasts, skinless, boneless, cubed
- 2 tablespoons olive oil
- 2 cups broccoli florets
- 1 teaspoon smoked paprika
- 1 teaspoon rosemary, dried
- 1 teaspoon oregano, dried
- 1 cup chicken stock
- 1 cup parmesan, grated
- A pinch of salt and black pepper

Directions:
Heat up a pan with the oil over medium heat, add the chicken and brown it for 5 minutes. Transfer this to a baking dish, add the broccoli and the other ingredients except the cheese and toss. Sprinkle the cheese on top, introduce the pan in the oven and bake at 370 degrees F for 30 minute Divide between plates and serve.

Nutrition: calories 250, fat 5, fiber 4, carbs 6, protein 25

Chicken, Tomatoes and Green Beans
The taste is so amazing!

Preparation time: 10 minutes
Cooking time: 35 minutes
Servings: 4

Ingredients:

- 2 tablespoons olive oil
- 1 pound chicken breast, skinless, boneless and cubed
- 1 cup cherry tomatoes, halved
- 1 celery stalks, chopped
- ½ pound green beans, trimmed and halved
- 1 cup tomato passata
- 1 cup mozzarella, shredded
- A pinch of salt and black pepper
- 1 tablespoon cilantro, chopped

Directions:

Heat up a pan with the oil over medium heat, add the chicken and the celery and cook for 5 minutes. Add the green beans and the other ingredients except the cheese, toss and cook for 5 minutes more. Sprinkle the cheese on top, introduce in the oven and bake at 380 degrees F for 25 minutes. Divide the mix between plates and serve.

Nutrition: calories 400, fat 23, fiber 5, carbs 5, protein 30

Ground Chicken and Spicy Tomatoes
These are even better than you can imagine!

Preparation time: 10 minutes
Cooking time: 30 minutes
Servings: 4

Ingredients:

- 1 pound chicken breast, skinless, boneless and ground
- 2 spring onions, chopped
- 1 tablespoon olive oil
- 1 teaspoon hot paprika
- 1 teaspoon chili powder
- ½ pound cherry tomatoes, halved
- 1 cup chicken stock
- 1 tablespoon cilantro, chopped

Directions:

Heat up a pan with the oil over medium heat, add the meat and the onions, stir and brown for 5 minutes. Add the rest of the ingredients, toss, bring to a simmer and cook over medium heat for 20 minutes more. Divide everything into bowls and serve.

Nutrition: calories 360, fat 32, fiber 2, carbs 7, protein 20

Unbelievable Chicken Dish

It's so yummy! We adore this dish and you will too!

Preparation time: 10 minutes
Cooking time: 50 minutes
Servings: 4

Ingredients:

- 3 pounds chicken breasts
- 2 ounces muenster cheese, cubed
- 2 ounces cream cheese
- 4 ounces cheddar cheese, cubed
- 2 ounces provolone cheese, cubed
- 1 zucchini, shredded
- Salt and black pepper to the taste
- 1 teaspoon garlic, minced
- ½ cup bacon, cooked and crumbled

Directions:

Season zucchini with salt and pepper, leave aside few minutes, squeeze well and transfer to a bowl. dd bacon, garlic, more salt and pepper, cream cheese, cheddar cheese, muenster cheese and provolone cheese and stir. Cut slits into chicken breasts, season with salt and pepper and stuff with zucchini and cheese mix. Place on a lined baking sheet, introduce in the oven at 400 degrees F and bake for 45 minutes. Divide on plates and serve.

Nutrition: calories 455, fat 20, fiber 0, carbs 2, protein 57

Delicious Crusted Chicken

You will soon end up recommending this amazing keto dish to everyone!

Preparation time: 10 minutes
Cooking time: 35 minutes
Servings: 4

Ingredients:

- 4 bacon slices, cooked and crumbled
- 4 chicken breasts, skinless and boneless
- 1 tablespoon water
- ½ cup avocado oil
- 1 egg, whisked
- Salt and black pepper to the taste
- 1 cup asiago cheese, shredded
- ¼ teaspoon garlic powder
- 1 cup parmesan cheese, grated

Directions:

In a bowl, mix parmesan cheese with garlic, salt and pepper and stir. Put whisked egg in another bowl and mix with the water. Season chicken with salt and pepper and dip each pieces into egg and then into cheese mix. Heat up a pan with the oil over medium high heat, add chicken breasts, cook until they are golden on both sides and transfer to a baking pan. Introduce in the oven at 350 degrees F and bake for 20 minutes. Top chicken with bacon and asiago cheese, introduce in the oven, turn on broiler and broil for a couple of minutes. Serve hot.

Nutrition: calories 400, fat 22, fiber 1, carbs 1, protein 47

Cheesy Chicken
Your friends will ask for more!

Preparation time: 10 minutes
Cooking time: 30 minutes
Servings: 4
Ingredients:

- 1 zucchini, chopped
- Salt and black pepper to the taste
- 1 teaspoon garlic powder
- 1 tablespoon avocado oil
- 2 chicken breasts,
- 1 tomato, chopped
- ½ teaspoon oregano, dried
- ⅓ teaspoon basil, dried
- ½ cup mozzarella cheese

Directions:

Season chicken with salt, pepper and garlic powder. Heat up a pan with the oil over medium heat, add chicken slices, brown on all sides and transfer them to a baking dish. Heat up the pan again over medium heat, add zucchini, oregano, tomato, basil, salt and pepper, stir, cook for 2 minutes and pour over chicken. Introduce in the oven at 325 degrees F and bake for 20 minutes. Spread mozzarella over chicken, introduce in the oven again and bake for 5 minutes more. Divide on plates and serve.

Nutrition: calories 235, fat 4, fiber 1, carbs 2, protein 35

Orange Chicken
The combination is absolutely delicious!

Preparation time: 10 minutes
Cooking time: 15 minutes
Servings: 4
Ingredients:

- 2 pounds chicken thighs, skinless, boneless and cut into pieces
- Salt and black pepper to the taste
- 3 tablespoons coconut oil
- ¼ cup coconut flour

For the sauce:

- 2 tablespoons fish sauce
- 1 and ½ teaspoons orange extract
- 1 tablespoon ginger, grated
- ¼ cup orange juice
- 2 teaspoons stevia
- 1 tablespoon orange zest
- ¼ teaspoon sesame seeds
- 2 tablespoons scallions, chopped
- ½ teaspoon coriander, ground
- 1 cup water
- ¼ teaspoon red pepper flakes
- 2 tablespoons gluten free soy sauce

Directions:

In a bowl, mix coconut flour and salt and pepper and stir. Add chicken pieces and toss to coat well. Heat up a pan with the oil over medium heat, add chicken, cook until they are golden on both sides and transfer to a bowl. In your blender, mix orange juice with ginger, fish sauce, soy sauce, stevia, orange extract, water and coriander and blend well. Pour this into a pan and heat up over medium heat. Add chicken, stir and cook for 2 minutes. Add sesame seeds, orange zest, scallions and pepper flakes, stir cook for 2 minutes and take off heat. Divide on plates and serve.

Nutrition: calories 423, fat 20, fiber 5, carbs 6, protein 45

Chicken Pie

This pie is so delicious!

Preparation time: 10 minutes
Cooking time: 45 minutes
Servings: 4
Ingredients:

- ½ cup yellow onion, chopped
- 3 tablespoons ghee
- ½ cup carrots, chopped
- 3 garlic cloves, minced
- Salt and black pepper to the taste
- ¾ cup heavy cream
- ½ cup chicken stock
- 12 ounces chicken, cubed
- 2 tablespoons Dijon mustard
- ¾ cup cheddar cheese, shredded

For the dough:

- ¾ cup almond flour
- 3 tablespoons cream cheese
- 1 and ½ cup mozzarella cheese
- 1 egg
- 1 teaspoon onion powder
- 1 teaspoon garlic powder
- 1 teaspoon Italian seasoning

Directions:

Heat up a pan with the ghee over medium heat, add onion, carrots, garlic, salt and pepper, stir and cook for 5 minutes. Add chicken, stir and cook for 3 minutes more. Add heavy cream, stock, salt, pepper and mustard, stir and cook for 7 minutes more. Add cheddar cheese, stir well, take off heat and keep warm. Meanwhile, in a bowl, mix mozzarella with cream cheese, stir and heat up in your microwave for 1 minute. Add garlic powder, Italian seasoning, salt, pepper, onion powder, flour and egg and stir well. Knead your dough very well, divide into 4 pieces and flatten each into a circle. Divide chicken mix into 4 ramekins, top each with a dough circle, introduce in the oven at 375 degrees F for 25 minutes. Serve your chicken pies warm.

Nutrition: calories 600, fat 54, fiber 14, carbs 10, protein 45

Bacon Wrapped Chicken

The flavors will hypnotize you for sure!

Preparation time: 10 minutes
Cooking time: 35 minutes
Servings: 4
Ingredients:

- 1 tablespoon chives, chopped
- 8 ounces cream cheese
- 2 pounds chicken breasts, skinless and boneless
- 12 bacon slices
- Salt and black pepper to the taste

Directions:

Heat up a pan over medium heat, add bacon, cook until it's half done, transfer to paper towels and drain grease. In a bowl, mix cream cheese with salt, pepper and chives and stir. Use a meat tenderizer to flatten chicken breasts well, divide cream cheese mix, roll them up and wrap each in a cooked bacon slice. Arrange wrapped chicken breasts into a baking dish, introduce in the oven at 375 degrees F and bake for 30 minutes. Divide on plates and serve.

Nutrition: calories 700, fat 45, fiber 4, carbs 5, protein 45

So Delicious Chicken Wings

You will fall in love with this keto dish and you will make it over and over again!

Preparation time: 10 minutes
Cooking time: 55 minutes
Servings: 4
Ingredients:

- 3 pounds chicken wings
- Salt and black pepper to the taste
- 3 tablespoons coconut aminos
- 2 teaspoons white vinegar
- 3 tablespoons rice vinegar
- 3 tablespoons stevia
- ¼ cup scallions, chopped
- ½ teaspoon xantham gum
- 5 dried chilies, chopped

Directions:

Spread chicken wings on a lined baking sheet, season with salt and pepper, introduce in the oven at 375 degrees F and bake for 45 minutes. Meanwhile, heat up a small pan over medium heat, add white vinegar, rice vinegar, coconut aminos, stevia, xantham gum, scallions and chilies, stir well, bring to a boil, cook for 2 minutes and take off heat. Dip chicken wings into this sauce, arrange them all on the baking sheet again and bake for 10 minutes more. Serve them hot.

Nutrition: calories 415, fat 23, fiber 3, carbs 2, protein 27

Chicken In Creamy Sauce

Trust us! This keto recipe is here to impress you!

Preparation time: 10 minutes
Cooking time: 1 hour and 10 minutes
Servings: 4
Ingredients:

- 8 chicken thighs
- Salt and black pepper to the taste
- 1 yellow onion, chopped
- 1 tablespoon coconut oil
- 4 bacon strips, chopped
- 4 garlic cloves, minced
- 10 ounces cremimi mushrooms, halved
- 2 cups white chardonnay wine
- 1 cup whipping cream
- A handful parsley, chopped

Directions:

Heat up a pan with the oil over medium heat, add bacon, stir, cook until it's crispy, take off heat and transfer to paper towels. Heat up the pan with the bacon fat over medium heat, add chicken pieces, season them with salt and pepper, cook until they brown and also transfer to paper towels. Heat up the pan again over medium heat, add onions, stir and cook for 6 minutes. Add garlic, stir, cook for 1 minute and transfer next to bacon pieces. Return pan to stove and heat up again over medium temperature. Add mushrooms stir and cook them for 5 minutes. Return chicken, bacon, garlic and onion to pan. Add wine, stir, bring to a boil, reduce heat and simmer fro 40 minutes. Add parsley and cream, stir and cook for 10 minutes more. Divide on plates and serve.

Nutrition: calories 340, fat 10, fiber 7, carbs 4, protein 24

Delightful Chicken
It's a delicious and textured keto poultry dish!

Preparation time: 10 minutes
Cooking time: 1 hour
Servings: 4

Ingredients:
- 6 chicken breasts, skinless and boneless
- Salt and black pepper to the taste
- ¼ cup jalapenos, chopped
- 5 bacon slices, chopped
- 8 ounces cream cheese
- ¼ cup yellow onion, chopped
- ½ cup mayonnaise
- ½ cup parmesan, grated
- 1 cup cheddar cheese, grated

For the topping:
- 2 ounces pork skins, crushed
- 4 tablespoons melted ghee
- ½ cup parmesan

Directions:

Arrange chicken breasts in a baking dish, season with salt and pepper, introduce in the oven at 425 degrees F and bake for 40 minutes. Meanwhile, heat up a pan over medium heat, add bacon, stir, cook until it's crispy and transfer to a plate. Heat up the pan again over medium heat, add onions, stir and cook for 4 minutes. Take off heat, add bacon, jalapeno, cream cheese, mayo, cheddar cheese and ½ cup parm and stir well. Spread this over chicken. In a bowl, mix pork skin with ghee and ½ cup parm and stir. Spread this over chicken as well, introduce in the oven and bake for 15 minutes more. Serve hot.

Nutrition: calories 340, fat 12, fiber 2, carbs 5, protein 20

Tasty Chicken And Sour Cream Sauce
You've got to learn how to make this tasty keto dish! It's so tasty!

Preparation time: 10 minutes
Cooking time: 40 minutes
Servings: 4

Ingredients:
- 4 chicken thighs
- Salt and black pepper to the taste
- 1 teaspoon onion powder
- ¼ cup sour cream
- 2 tablespoons sweet paprika

Directions:

In a bowl, mix paprika with salt, pepper and onion powder and stir. Season chicken pieces with this paprika mix, arrange them on a lined baking sheet and bake in the oven at 400 degrees F for 40 minutes. Divide chicken on plates and leave aside for now. Pour juices from the pan into a bowl and add sour cream. Stir this sauce very well and drizzle over chicken.

Nutrition: calories 384, fat 31, fiber 2, carbs 1, protein 33

Tasty Chicken Stroganoff

Have you heard about this keto recipe? It seems it's amazing!

Preparation time: 10 minutes
Cooking time: 4 hours and 10 minutes
Servings: 4
Ingredients:

- 2 garlic cloves, minced
- 8 ounces mushrooms, roughly chopped
- ¼ teaspoon celery seeds, ground
- 1 cup chicken stock
- 1 cup coconut milk
- 1 yellow onion, chopped
- 1 pound chicken breasts, cut into medium pieces
- 1 and ½ teaspoons thyme, dried
- 2 tablespoons parsley, chopped
- Salt and black pepper to the tasted
- 4 zucchinis, cut with a spiralizer

Directions:

Put chicken in your slow cooker. Add salt, pepper, onion, garlic, mushrooms, coconut milk, celery seeds, stock, half of the parsley and thyme. Stir, cover and cook on High for 4 hours. Uncover pot, add more salt and pepper if needed and the rest of the parsley and stir. Heat up a pan with water over medium heat, add some salt, bring to a boil, add zucchini pasta, cook for 1 minute and drain. Divide on plates, add chicken mix on top and serve.

Nutrition: calories 364, fat 22, fiber 2, carbs 4, protein 24

Tasty Chicken Gumbo

Oh..you are going to love this!

Preparation time: 10 minutes
Cooking time: 7 hours
Servings: 5
Ingredients:

- 2 sausages, sliced
- 3 chicken breasts, cubed
- 2 tablespoons oregano, dried
- 2 bell peppers, chopped
- 1 small yellow onion, chopped
- 28 ounces canned tomatoes, chopped
- 3 tablespoons thyme, dried
- 2 tablespoons garlic powder
- 2 tablespoons mustard powder
- 1 teaspoon cayenne powder
- 1 tablespoons chili powder
- Salt and black pepper to the taste
- 6 tablespoons Creole seasoning

Directions:

In your slow cooker, mix sausages with chicken pieces, salt, pepper, bell peppers, oregano, onion, thyme, garlic powder, mustard powder, tomatoes, cayenne, chili and Creole seasoning. Cover and cook on Low for 7 hours. Uncover pot again, stir gumbo and divide into bowls. Serve hot.

Nutrition: calories 360, fat 23, fiber 2, carbs 6, protein 23

Tender Chicken Thighs
You'll see what we're talking about!

Preparation time: 10 minutes
Cooking time: 45 minutes
Servings: 4

Ingredients:
- 3 tablespoons ghee
- 8 ounces mushrooms, sliced
- 2 tablespoons gruyere cheese, grated
- Salt and black pepper to the taste
- 2 garlic cloves, minced
- 6 chicken thighs, skin and bone-in

Directions:
Heat up a pan with 1 tablespoon ghee over medium heat, add chicken thighs, season with salt and pepper, cook for 3 minutes on each side and arrange them into a baking dish. Heat up the pan again with the rest of the ghee over medium heat, add garlic, stir and cook for 1 minute. Add mushrooms and stir well. Add salt and pepper, stir and cook for 10 minutes. Spoon these over chicken, sprinkle cheese, introduce in the oven at 350 degrees F and bake for 30 minutes. Turn oven to broiler and broil everything for a couple more minutes. Divide on plates and serve.

Nutrition: calories 340, fat 31, fiber 3, carbs 5, protein 64

Tasty Crusted Chicken
This is just perfect!

Preparation time: 10 minutes
Cooking time: 20 minutes
Servings: 4

Ingredients:
- 1 egg, whisked
- Salt and black pepper to the taste
- 3 tablespoons coconut oil
- 1 and ½ cups pecans, chopped
- 4 chicken breasts
- Salt and black pepper to the taste

Directions:
Put pecans in a bowl and the whisked egg in another. Season chicken, dip in egg and then in pecans. Heat up a pan with the oil over medium high heat, add chicken and cook until it's brown on both sides. Transfer chicken pieces to a baking sheet, introduce in the oven and bake at 350 degrees F for 10 minutes. Divide on plates and serve.

Nutrition: calories 320, fat 12, fiber 4, carbs 1, protein 30

Pepperoni Chicken Bake

It's impossible not to appreciate this great keto dish!

Preparation time: 10 minutes
Cooking time: 55 minutes
Servings: 6

Ingredients:

- 14 ounces low carb pizza sauce
- 1 tablespoon coconut oil
- 4 medium chicken breasts, skinless and boneless
- Salt and black pepper to the taste
- 1 teaspoon oregano, dried
- 6 ounces mozzarella, sliced
- 1 teaspoon garlic powder
- 2 ounces pepperoni, sliced

Directions:

Put pizza sauce in a small pot, bring to a boil over medium heat, simmer for 20 minutes and take off heat. In a bowl, mix chicken with salt, pepper, garlic powder and oregano and stir. Heat up a pan with the coconut oil over medium high heat, add chicken pieces, cook for 2 minutes on each side and transfer them to a baking dish. Add mozzarella slices on top, spread sauce, top with pepperoni slices, introduce in the oven at 400 degrees F and bake for 30 minutes. Divide on plates and serve.

Nutrition: calories 320, fat 10, fiber 6, carbs 3, protein 27

Fried Chicken

It's a very simple dish you will like!

Preparation time: 24 hours
Cooking time: 20 minutes
Servings: 4

Ingredients:

- 3 chicken breasts, cut in strips
- 4 ounces pork rinds, crushed
- 2 cups coconut oil
- 16 ounces jarred pickle juice
- 2 eggs, whisked

Directions:

In a bowl, mix chicken breast pieces with pickle juice, stir, cover and keep in the fridge for 24 hours. Put eggs in a bowl and pork rinds in another one. Dip chicken pieces in egg and then in rinds and coat well. Heat up a pan with the oil over medium high heat, add chicken pieces, fry them for 3 minutes on each side, transfer them to paper towels and drain grease. Serve with a keto aioli sauce on the side.

Nutrition: calories 260, fat 5, fiber 1, carbs 2, protein 20

Chicken Calzone
This special calzone is so delicious!

Preparation time: 10 minutes
Cooking time: 1 hour
Servings: 12

Ingredients:
- 2 eggs
- 1 keto pizza crust
- ½ cup parmesan, grated
- 1 pound chicken breasts, skinless, boneless and each sliced in halves
- ½ cup keto marinara sauce
- 1 teaspoon Italian seasoning
- 1 teaspoon onion powder
- 1 teaspoon garlic powder
- Salt and black pepper to the taste
- ¼ cup flaxseed, ground
- 8 ounces provolone cheese

Directions:
In a bowl, mix Italian seasoning with onion powder, garlic powder, salt, pepper, flaxseed and parmesan and stir well. In another bowl, mix eggs with a pinch of salt and pepper and whisk well. Dip chicken pieces in eggs and then in seasoning mix, place all pieces on a lined baking sheet and bake in the oven at 350 degrees F for 30 minutes. Put pizza crust dough on a lined baking sheet and spread half of the provolone cheese on half. Take chicken out of the oven, chop and spread over provolone cheese. Add marinara sauce and then the rest of the cheese. Cover all these with the other half of the dough and shape your calzone. Seal its edges, introduce in the oven at 350 degrees F and bake for 20 minuets more. Leave calzone to cool down before slicing and serving.

Nutrition: calories 340, fat 8, fiber 2, carbs 6, protein 20

Mexican Chicken Soup
It's very simple to make a tasty keto chicken soup! Try this one!

Preparation time: 10 minutes
Cooking time: 4 hours
Servings: 6

Ingredients:
- 1 and ½ pounds chicken tights, skinless, boneless and cubed
- 15 ounces chicken stock
- 15 ounces canned chunky salsa
- 8 ounces Monterey jack

Directions:
In your slow cooker, mix chicken with stock, salsa and cheese, stir, cover and cook on High for 4 hours. Uncover pot, stir soup, divide into bowls and serve.

Nutrition: calories 400, fat 22, fiber 3, carbs 6, protein 38

Simple Chicken Stir Fry

It's a keto friendly recipe you should really try soon!

Preparation time: 10 minutes
Cooking time: 12 minutes
Servings: 2

Ingredients:

- 2 chicken thighs, skinless, boneless cut in thin strips
- 1 tablespoon sesame oil
- 1 teaspoon red pepper flakes
- 1 teaspoon onion powder
- 1 tablespoon ginger, grated
- ¼ cup tamari sauce
- ½ teaspoon garlic powder
- ½ cup water
- 1 tablespoon stevia
- ½ teaspoon xantham gum
- ½ cup scallions, chopped
- 2 cups broccoli florets

Directions:

Heat up a pan with the oil over medium high heat, add chicken and ginger, stir and cook for 3 minutes. Add water, tamari sauce, onion powder, garlic powder, stevia, pepper flakes and xantham gum, stir and cook for 5 minutes. Add broccoli and scallions, stir, cook for 2 minutes more and divide on plates. Serve hot.

Nutrition: calories 210, fat 10, fiber 3, carbs 5, protein 20

Spinach And Artichoke Chicken

The combination is really exceptional!

Preparation time: 10 minutes
Cooking time: 50 minutes
Servings: 4

Ingredients:

- 4 ounces cream cheese
- 4 chicken breasts
- 10 ounces canned artichoke hearts, chopped
- 10 ounces spinach
- ½ cup parmesan, grated
- 1 tablespoon dried onion
- 1 tablespoon garlic, dried
- Salt and black pepper to the taste
- 4 ounces mozzarella, shredded

Directions:

Place chicken breasts on a lined baking sheet, season with salt and pepper, introduce in the oven at 400 degrees F and bake for 30 minutes. In a bowl, mix artichokes with onion, cream cheese, parmesan, spinach, garlic, salt and pepper and stir. Take chicken out of the oven, cut each piece in the middle, divide artichokes mix, sprinkle mozzarella, introduce in the oven at 400 degrees F and bake for 15 minutes more. Serve hot.

Nutrition: calories 450, fat 23, fiber 1, carbs 3, protein 39

Chicken Meatloaf

This is a special keto recipe we want to share with you!

Preparation time: 10 minutes
Cooking time: 40 minutes
Servings: 8
Ingredients:

- 1 cup keto marinara sauce
- 2 pound chicken meat, ground
- 2 tablespoons parsley, chopped
- 4 garlic cloves, minced
- 2 teaspoons onion powder
- 2 teaspoons Italian seasoning

- ½ cup ricotta cheese
- 1 cup parmesan, grated
- 1 cup mozzarella, shredded
- 2 teaspoons chives, chopped
- 2 tablespoons parsley, chopped
- 1 garlic clove, minced

For the filling:

Directions:

In a bowl, mix chicken with half of the marinara sauce, salt, pepper, Italian seasoning, 4 garlic cloves, onion powder and 2 tablespoons parsley and stir well. In another bowl, mix ricotta with half of the parmesan, half of the mozzarella, chives, 1 garlic clove, salt, pepper and 2 tablespoons parsley and stir well. Put half of the chicken mix into a loaf pan and spread evenly. Add cheese filling and also spread. Top with the rest of the meat and spread again. Introduce meatloaf in the oven at 400 degrees F and bake for 20 minutes. Take meatloaf out of the oven, spread the rest of the marinara sauce, the rest of the parmesan and mozzarella and bake for 20 minutes more. Leave meatloaf to cool down, slice, divide on plates and serve.

Nutrition: calories 273, fat 14, fiber 1, carbs 4, protein 28

Delicious Whole Chicken

Cook this keto dish for a special occasion!

Preparation time: 10 minutes
Cooking time: 40 minutes
Servings: 12
Ingredients:

- 1 whole chicken
- ½ teaspoon onion powder
- ½ teaspoon garlic powder
- Salt and black pepper to the taste

- 2 tablespoons coconut oil
- 1 teaspoon Italian seasoning
- 1 and ½ cups chicken stock
- 2 teaspoons guar guar

Directions:

Rub chicken with half of the oil, garlic powder, salt, pepper, Italian seasoning and onion powder. Put the rest of the oil into an instant pot and add chicken to the pot. Add stock, cover pot and cook on High for 40 minutes. Transfer chicken to a platter and leave aside for now. Set the instant pot on Sauté mode, add guar guar, stir and cook until it thickens. Pour sauce over chicken and serve.

Nutrition: calories 450, fat 30, fiber 1, carbs 1, protein 34

Chicken And Green Onion Sauce

Tell all your friends about this keto dish!

Preparation time: 10 minutes
Cooking time: 27 minutes
Servings: 4

Ingredients:

- 2 tablespoons ghee
- 1 green onion, chopped
- 4 chicken breast halves, skinless and boneless
- Salt and black pepper to the taste
- 8 ounces sour cream

Directions:

Heat up a pan with the ghee over medium high heat, add chicken pieces, season with salt and pepper, cover, reduce heat and simmer for 10 minutes. Uncover pan, turn chicken pieces and cook them covered for 10 minutes more Add green onions, stir and cook for 2 minutes more. Take off heat, add more salt and pepper if needed, add sour cream, stir well, cover pan and leave aside for 5 minutes. Stir again, divide on plates and serve.

Nutrition: calories 200, fat 7, fiber 2, carbs 1, protein 8

Chicken Stuffed Mushrooms

It's a simple recipe you will like for sure!

Preparation time: 10 minutes
Cooking time: 10 minutes
Servings: 6

Ingredients:

- 16 ounces button mushroom caps
- 4 ounces cream cheese
- ¼ cup carrot, chopped
- 1 teaspoon ranch seasoning mix
- 4 tablespoons hot sauce
- ¾ cup blue cheese, crumbled
- ¼ cup red onion, chopped
- ½ cup chicken meat, already cooked and chopped
- Salt and black pepper to the taste
- Cooking spray

Directions:

In a bowl, mix cream cheese with blue cheese, hot sauce, ranch seasoning, salt, pepper, chicken, carrot and red onion and stir. Stuff each mushroom cap with this mix, place them all on a lined baking sheet, spray with cooking spray, introduce in the oven at 425 degrees F and bake for 10 minutes. Divide on plates and serve them.

Nutrition: calories 200, fat 4, fiber 1, carbs 2, protein 7

Chicken Stuffed Avocado

You will have to share this with all your friends!

Preparation time: 10 minutes
Cooking time: 0 minutes
Servings: 2

Ingredients:

- 2 avocados, cut in halves and pitted
- ¼ cup mayonnaise
- 1 teaspoon thyme, dried
- 2 tablespoons cream cheese
- 1 and ½ cups chicken, cooked and shredded
- Salt and black pepper to the taste
- ¼ teaspoon cayenne pepper
- ½ teaspoon onion powder
- ½ teaspoon garlic powder
- 1 teaspoon paprika
- Salt and black pepper to the taste
- 2 tablespoons lemon juice

Directions:

Scoop the insides of your avocado halves and put flesh in a bowl. Leave avocado cups aside for now. Add chicken to avocado flesh and stir. Also add mayo, thyme, cream cheese, cayenne, onion, garlic, paprika, salt, pepper and lemon juice and stir well. Stuff avocados with chicken mix and serve.

Nutrition: calories 230, fat 40, fiber 11, carbs 5, protein 24

Delicious Balsamic Chicken

It's an easy dish you can make today!

Preparation time: 10 minutes
Cooking time: 20 minutes
Servings: 4

Ingredients:

- 3 tablespoons coconut oil
- 2 pounds chicken breasts, skinless and boneless
- 3 garlic cloves, minced
- Salt and black pepper to the taste
- 1 cup chicken stock
- 3 tablespoons stevia
- ½ cup balsamic vinegar
- 1 tomato, thinly sliced
- 6 mozzarella slices
- Some chopped basil for serving

Directions:

Heat up a pan with the oil over medium high heat, add chicken pieces, season with salt and pepper, cook until they brown on both sides and reduce heat. Add garlic, vinegar, stock and stevia, stir, increase heat again and cook for 10 minutes. Transfer chicken breasts to a lined baking sheet, arrange mozzarella slices on top, then top with basil. Broil in the oven over medium heat until cheese melts and then arrange tomato slices over chicken pieces. Divide on plates and serve.

Nutrition: calories 240, fat 12, fiber 1, carbs 4, protein 27

Chicken Pasta

It's a very great dinner idea! This keto dish is superb!

Preparation time: 10 minutes
Cooking time: 30 minutes
Servings: 4
Ingredients:

- 2 tablespoons ghee
- 1 teaspoon garlic, minced
- 1 pound chicken cutlets
- 1 teaspoon Cajun seasoning
- ¼ cup scallions, chopped
- ½ cup tomatoes, chopped
- ½ cup chicken stock
- ¼ cup whipping cream
- ½ cup cheddar cheese, grated
- 1 ounce cream cheese
- ¼ cup cilantro, chopped
- *For the pasta:*
- 4 ounces cream cheese
- 8 eggs

Directions:

Heat up a pan with 1 tablespoon ghee over medium heat, add chicken cutlets, season with some of the Cajun seasoning, cook for 2 minutes on each side and transfer to a plate. Heat up the pan with the rest of the ghee over medium heat, add garlic, stir and cook for 2 minutes. Add tomatoes, stir and cook for 2 minutes more. Add stock and the rest of the Cajun seasoning, stir and cook for 5 minutes. Add whipping cream, cheddar cheese, 1 ounce cream cheese, salt, pepper, scallions and cilantro, stir well, cook for 2 minutes more and take off heat. Meanwhile, in your blender, mix 4 ounces cream cheese with eggs, salt, pepper and garlic powder and pulse well. Pour this into a lined baking sheet, leave aside for 5 minutes and then bake in the oven at 325 degrees F for 10 minutes. Leave pasta sheet to cool down, transfer to a cutting board, roll and cut into medium slices. Divide pasta on plates, top with chicken mix and serve.

Nutrition: calories 345, fat 34, fiber 4, carbs 4, protein 39

Peanut Grilled Chicken

It's a Thai keto recipe worth trying!

Preparation time: 10 minutes
Cooking time: 20 minutes
Servings: 8
Ingredients:

- 2 and ½ pounds chicken thighs and drumsticks
- 1 tablespoon coconut aminos
- 1 tablespoon apple cider vinegar
- A pinch of red pepper flakes
- **Directions:**
- ½ teaspoon ginger, ground
- 1/3 cup peanut butter
- 1 garlic clove, minced
- ½ cup warm water

In your blender mix peanut butter with water, aminos, salt, pepper, pepper flakes, ginger, garlic and vinegar and blend well. Pat dry chicken pieces, arrange them in a pan and pour the peanut butter marinade over it. Toss to coat and keep in the fridge for 1 hour. Place chicken pieces skin side down on your preheated grill over medium high heat, cook for 10 minutes, flip, brush with some of the marinade and cook them for 10 minutes more. Divide on plates and serve.

Nutrition: calories 375, fat 12, fiber 1, carbs 3, protein 42

Simple Chicken Stew

It's so easy to make a delicious and simple keto chicken stew!

Preparation time: 10 minutes
Cooking time: 2 hours
Servings: 4
Ingredients:

- 2 carrots, chopped
- 2 celery sticks, chopped
- 2 cups chicken stock
- 1 small onion, chopped
- 28 ounces chicken thighs, skinless, boneless and cut in medium pieces
- 3 garlic cloves, minced
- ½ teaspoon rosemary, dried
- 1 cup spinach
- ½ teaspoon oregano, dried
- ¼ teaspoon thyme, dried
- ½ cup heavy cream
- Salt and black pepper to the taste
- A pinch of xantham gum

Directions:

In your slow cooker, mix chicken with stock, celery, carrots, onion, garlic, rosemary, thyme, oregano, some salt and pepper, stir, cover and cook on High for 2 hours. Add more salt and pepper to the taste, spinach and heavy cream and stir. Add xantham gum, stir and cook for 10 minutes more. Divide into bowls and serve.

Nutrition: calories 224, fat 11, fiber 4, carbs 6, protein 23

Chicken And Veggie Stew

Why don't you try something special for a change? This creamy keto stew is divine!

Preparation time: 10 minutes
Cooking time: 30 minutes
Servings: 6
Ingredients:

- 2 cups whipping cream
- 40 ounces rotisserie chicken pieces, boneless, skinless and shredded
- 3 tablespoons ghee
- ½ cup yellow onion, chopped
- ¾ cup red peppers, chopped
- 29 ounces canned chicken stock
- Salt and black pepper to the taste
- 1 bay leaf
- 8 ounces mushrooms, chopped
- 1 cup green snap beans
- 17 ounces asparagus, trimmed
- 3 teaspoons thyme, chopped

Directions:

Heat up a pan with the cream over medium heat, bring to a simmer and cook until it's reduced for 7 minutes. Meanwhile, heat up a pan with the ghee over medium heat, add onion and peppers, stir and cook for 3 minutes. Add stock, bay leaf, some salt and pepper, bring to a boil and simmer for 10 minutes. Add asparagus, green beans and mushrooms, stir and cook for 7 minutes. Add chicken pieces, stir and cook for 3 minutes more. Add cream, thyme, salt and pepper to the taste, stir, discard bay leaf, divide stew into bowls and serve.

Nutrition: calories 500, fat 27, fiber 3, carbs 4, protein 47

Ketogenic Meat Recipes

Pork and Tomatoes
> *This pork dish will surprise you for sure!*

Preparation time: 10 minutes
Cooking time: 45 minutes
Servings: 4

Ingredients:
- 2 tablespoons olive oil
- 1 pound pork loin, cubed
- 2 cups cherry tomatoes, halved
- 2 shallots, chopped
- 1 tablespoon lime juice
- 1 cup beef stock
- 1 teaspoon sweet paprika
- 1 teaspoon cumin, ground
- 1 tablespoon cilantro, chopped
- A pinch of salt and black pepper

Directions:
Heat up a pan with the oil over medium heat, add the meat and shallots and brown for 5 minutes. Add the rest of the ingredients, toss, introduce in the oven and bake at 390 degrees F for 40 minutes. Divide everything between plates and serve.

Nutrition: calories 361, fat 23.3, fiber 1.4, carbs 5, protein 32.7

Garlic Pork and Zucchinis
> *Try this keto dish really soon!*

Preparation time: 10 minutes
Cooking time: 35 minutes
Servings: 4

Ingredients:
- 2 tablespoons avocado oil
- 2 spring onions, chopped
- 1 pound pork stew meat, cubed
- 1 zucchini, cubed
- 3 garlic cloves, minced
- 1 cup tomato passata
- 1 cup cilantro, chopped
- A pinch of salt and black pepper
- 1 tablespoon oregano, chopped

Directions:
Heat up a pan with the oil over medium heat, add the garlic and the spring onions, stir and sauté for 2 minutes. Add the meat and brown for 5 minutes more. Add the rest of the ingredients, toss, bring to a simmer and cook over medium heat for 20 minutes more. Divide everything into bowls and serve.

Nutrition: calories 274, fat 12.1, fiber 2.2, carbs 5.2, protein 34.9

Balsamic Pork Chops

These pork chops are all you need to end this day!

Preparation time: 10 minutes
Cooking time: 20 minutes
Servings: 4

Ingredients:
- 4 pork chops
- 2 tablespoons olive oil
- 3 garlic cloves, minced
- 1 red onion, chopped
- 1 teaspoon nutmeg, ground
- 1 tablespoon balsamic vinegar
- 1 tablespoon rosemary, chopped

Directions:
Heat up a pan with the oil over medium heat, add the garlic and the pork chops and brown for 3 minutes on each side. Add the onion, and cook for 4 minutes more. Add the rest of the ingredients, toss, cook over medium heat for 10 minutes more, divide between plates and serve with a side salad.

Nutrition: calories 337, fat 27.3, fiber 1.1, carbs 4.1, protein 18.5

Rosemary Pork

You must pay attention and learn how to make this tasty keto dish!

Preparation time: 10 minutes
Cooking time: 30 minutes
Servings: 4

Ingredients:
- 1 pound pork stew meat, roughly cubed
- 1 tablespoon olive oil
- 2 shallots, chopped
- 1 tablespoon rosemary, chopped
- 1 cup beef stock
- 1 teaspoon sweet paprika
- A pinch of salt and black pepper

Directions:
Heat up a pan with the oil over medium heat, add the shallots and the meat and brown for 5 minutes. Add the rosemary and the other ingredients, toss, bring to a simmer and cook over medium heat for 25 minutes more. Divide the mix between plates and serve.

Nutrition: calories 279, fat 14.8, fiber 0.6, carbs 0.9, protein 34

Lime Pork

You will learn how to make this tasty keto dish really soon!

Preparation time: 10 minutes
Cooking time: 30 minutes
Servings: 4

Ingredients:

- 3 tablespoons olive oil
- 4 pork chops
- 1 cup beef stock
- A pinch of salt and black pepper
- 1 tablespoon lime juice
- 1 tablespoon lime zest, grated
- 2 tablespoons parsley, chopped

Directions:

Heat up a pan with the oil over medium high heat, add the pork and brown for 5 minutes. Add the stock and the other ingredients, toss, bring to a simmer and cook over medium heat for 25 minutes more. Divide everything between plates and serve.

Nutrition: calories 352, fat 30.5, fiber 0.2, carbs 0.4, protein 18.7

Cinnamon Pork

This simple keto dish will make you a star in the kitchen!

Preparation time: 10 minutes
Cooking time: 30 minutes
Servings: 4

Ingredients:

- 2 pounds pork stew meat, cubed
- 2 tablespoons olive oil
- 2 shallots, chopped
- 1 tablespoon cinnamon powder
- 1 tablespoon oregano, chopped
- 1 cup beef stock
- A pinch of salt and black pepper

Directions:

Heat up a pan with the oil over medium heat, add the shallots and the meat and brown for 5 minutes. Add the rest of the ingredients, toss, bring to a simmer and cook over medium heat for 25 minutes more. Divide the mix between plates and serve.

Nutrition: calories 552, fat 29.2, fiber 0.5, carbs 1.6, protein 67.3

Mustard Beef Mix

This is a keto dish that will impress you!

Preparation time: 10 minutes
Cooking time: 35 minutes
Servings: 4

Ingredients:

1 tablespoon avocado oil
1 pound beef stew meat, cubed
1 red onion, sliced
1 tablespoon rosemary, chopped

1 tablespoon mustard
1 cup beef stock
A pinch of salt and black pepper
1 teaspoon chili powder

Directions:

Heat up a pan with the oil over medium heat, add the meat and the onion and brown for 5 minutes. Add the rosemary and the other ingredients, toss, bring to a simmer and cook over medium heat for 30 minutes. Divide the mix into bowls and serve.

Nutrition: calories 430, fat 23, fiber 2, carbs 3, protein 45

Curry Beef

This will be so tender and delicious!

Preparation time: 10 minutes
Cooking time: 30 minutes
Servings: 4

Ingredients:

- 2 shallots, chopped
- 2 tablespoons avocado oil
- 1 pound beef stew meat, cubed
- 1 teaspoon curry powder

- 1 cup beef stock
- 1 cup coconut cream
- A pinch of salt and black pepper
- 1 tablespoon chives, chopped

Directions:

Heat up a pan with the oil over medium heat, add the shallots and the meat and brown for 5 minutes. Add the curry powder, toss and cook for 5 minutes more. Add the rest of the ingredients, bring to a simmer and cook over medium heat for 20 minutes more, stirring often. Divide the mix into bowls and serve.

Nutrition: calories 325, fat 18, fiber 1, carbs 5.6, protein 36

Ghee Pork Chops

This is going to be ready so fast!!

Preparation time: 10 minutes
Cooking time: 20 minutes
Servings: 4

Ingredients:

4 pork chops
1 shallot, chopped
3 tablespoons ghee, melted
1 tablespoon lime juice

1 tablespoon walnuts, chopped
A pinch of salt and black pepper
1 teaspoon lemon pepper

Directions:

Heat up a pan with the ghee over medium heat, add the shallot and the pork chops and brown for 3 minutes on each side. Add the rest of the ingredients, toss and cook over medium heat for 14 minutes more. Divide the mix between plates and serve.

Nutrition: calories 132, fat 5, fiber 1, carbs 1, protein 18

Pork with Olives

This great keto dinner idea will make you fell great!

Preparation time: 10 minutes
Cooking time: 30 minutes
Servings: 4

Ingredients:

1 pound pork stew meat, cubed
2 tablespoons ghee, melted
1 red onion, chopped
1 cup beef stock

1 cup black olives, pitted and halved
A pinch of salt and black pepper
2 garlic cloves, minced
1 tablespoon oregano, chopped

Directions:

Heat up a pan with the ghee over medium heat, add the onion and the meat and brown for 5 minutes. Add the rest of the ingredients, toss, cook over medium heat for 25 minutes more, divide into bowls and serve.

Nutrition: calories 165, fat 2, fiber 1, carbs 2, protein 26

Oregano Pork Chops

This is so yummy and simple to make at home!

Preparation time: 10 minutes
Cooking time: 36 minutes
Servings: 4

Ingredients:
- 4 pork chops
- 1 tablespoon oregano, chopped
- 2 tablespoons olive oil
- 1 cup tomato passata
- A pinch of salt and black pepper
- 1 tablespoon cilantro, chopped
- 2 tablespoons lime juice

Directions:

Heat up a pan with the oil over medium high heat, add the pork chops and the oregano, and brown for 3 minutes on each side. Add the rest of the ingredients, toss, bring to a simmer and cook over medium heat for 30 minutes. Divide the mix between plates and serve.

Nutrition: calories 210, fat 10, fiber 2, carbs 6, protein 19

Coconut Beef

These spicy pork chops will impress you for sure!

Preparation time: 10 minutes
Cooking time: 8 hours
Servings: 4

Ingredients:

- 1 pound beef stew meat, cubed
- 1 cup beef stock
- 1 tablespoon coconut oil
- 1 cup coconut cream
- 2 shallots, chopped
- 2 celery ribs, roughly chopped
- 2 garlic cloves, minced
- 1 tablespoon chili powder
- 2 teaspoons cumin, ground
- A pinch of salt and black pepper

Directions:

In your slow cooker, combine the meat with the stock and the other ingredients, put the lid on and cook on Low for 8 hours. Divide everything into bowls and serve.

Nutrition: calories 200, fat 8, fiber 1, carbs 5.3, protein 26

Beef, Tomato and Peppers

It will soon become your favorite keto dinner dish!

Preparation time: 10 minutes
Cooking time: 35 minutes
Servings: 4

Ingredients:

- 1 cup beef stock
- 1 pound beef stew meat, cubed
- 2 tomatoes, cubed
- 2 shallots, chopped
- 1 red bell pepper, cut into strips
- 1 yellow bell pepper, cut into strips
- 2 tablespoons olive oil
- ¼ teaspoon garlic powder
- A pinch of salt and black pepper

Directions:

Heat up a pan with the oil over medium high heat, add the meat and the shallots and brown for 5 minutes. Add the rest of the ingredients, bring to a simmer and cook over medium heat for 30 minutes more. Divide everything into bowls and serve.

Nutrition: calories 224, fat 15, fiber 1, carbs 3, protein 19

Pork Meatballs

This will be one of the best keto dishes you'll ever try!

Preparation time: 10 minutes
Cooking time: 10 minutes
Servings: 4

Ingredients:

- ½ cup almond meal
- 2 eggs
- 2 pounds pork stew meat, ground
- A pinch of salt and black pepper
- 2 tablespoons cilantro, chopped
- 2 garlic cloves, minced
- 2 shallots, chopped
- 2 tablespoons olive oil

Directions:

In a bowl, mix the pork with the eggs and the other ingredients except the oil, stir well and shape medium meatballs out of this mix. Heat up a pan with the oil over medium heat, add the meatballs, cook them for 5 minutes on each side, divide between plates and serve with a side salad.

Nutrition: calories 643, fat 37.1, fiber 1.5, carbs 3.3, protein 71.8

Herbed Beef Mix

It's so juicy and delicious!

Preparation time: 10 minutes
Cooking time: 30 minutes
Servings: 4

Ingredients:

- 2 pounds beef stew meat, cubed
- 2 tablespoons ghee, melted
- 2 spring onions, chopped
- 1 cup beef stock
- 1 tablespoon rosemary, chopped
- 1 tablespoon parsley, chopped
- tablespoon tarragon, chopped
- 1 teaspoon chili powder
- ½ teaspoon cumin, ground

Directions:

Heat up a pan with the ghee over medium heat, add the meat and spring onions and brown for 5 minutes. Add the rest of the ingredients, toss, bring to a simmer and cook over medium heat for 25 minutes more. Divide everything between plates and serve.

Nutrition: calories 700, fat 56, fiber 2, carbs 13.10, protein 70

Sage Beef

This looks so good and it tastes wonderful!

Preparation time: 10 minutes
Cooking time: 35 minutes
Servings: 4

Ingredients:

- 2 garlic cloves, minced
- 1 pound beef stew meat, cubed
- 2 tablespoons ghee, melted
- 2 shallots, chopped
- 1 celery stalks, chopped
- ½ cup beef stock
- A pinch of salt and black pepper
- 1 teaspoon cumin, ground
- 1 tablespoon sage, chopped

Directions:

Heat up a pan with the oil over medium high heat, add the garlic and the shallots and sauté for 5 minutes. Add the meat and brown for 5 minutes more. Add the rest of the ingredients, toss, bring to a simmer and cook over medium heat for 25 minutes.

Nutrition: calories 222, fat 10, fiber 2, carbs 8, protein 21

Beef Casserole
This is so special and of course, it's 100% keto!

Preparation time: 10 minutes
Cooking time: 35 minutes
Servings: 6

Ingredients:

- 1 pound beef stew meat, ground
- ¼ cup beef stock
- 2 shallots, chopped
- 2 tablespoons avocado oil
- A pinch of salt and black pepper
- ½ teaspoon red pepper flakes, crushed
- A pinch of cayenne pepper
- 1 cup cherry tomatoes, halved
- 1 cup zucchinis, cubed
- 1 cup parmesan, grated
- 1 tablespoon chives, chopped

Directions:

Heat up a pan with the oil over medium heat, add the meat and shallots and brown for 5 minutes. Add the tomatoes and the other ingredients except the parmesan and the chives, toss and cook for 5 minutes more. Sprinkle the cheese and chives on top, introduce the pan in the oven, bake at 375 degrees F for 25 minutes, divide between plates and serve hot.

Nutrition: calories 456, fat 35, fiber 3, carbs 4, protein 32

Thyme Beef and Leeks
It's always amazing to discover such interesting dishes!

Preparation time: 10 minutes
Cooking time: 35 minutes
Servings: 4

Ingredients:

- 2 pounds beef stew meat, cubed
- 2 tablespoons ghee, melted
- A pinch of salt and black pepper
- 2 leeks, sliced
- 1 cup beef stock
- 3 garlic cloves, minced
- 1 teaspoon oregano, dried
- 1 tablespoon thyme, chopped

Directions:

Heat up a pan with the ghee over medium high heat, add the leeks and garlic and sauté for 5 minutes. Add the meat and brown for 5 minutes more. Add the stock and the rest of the ingredients, bring to a simmer and cook over medium heat for 25 minutes more. Divide everything into bowls and serve.

Nutrition: calories 260, fat 7, fiber 2, carbs 4, protein 10

Coconut Pork and Celery
This is so delightful! You've got to try this really soon!

Preparation time: 10 minutes
Cooking time: 8 hours
Servings: 4

Ingredients:

- 2 shallots, chopped
- 2 pounds beef stew meat, cubed
- 1 tablespoon ghee, melted
- 1 cup tomato passata
- 2 jalapenos, minced
- 3 celery ribs, chopped
- 2 tablespoons coconut aminos
- A pinch of salt and black pepper
- A pinch of cayenne pepper
- 2 tablespoons cumin, ground
- 1 tablespoon oregano, chopped

Directions:

In your slow cooker, combine the meat with the shallots and the other ingredients, put the lid on and cook on Low for 8 hours. Divide everything between plates and serve.

Nutrition: calories 137, fat 6, fiber 2, carbs 5, protein 17

Pork and Mushroom Meatloaf
This will guarantee your success!

Preparation time: 10 minutes
Cooking time: 50 minutes
Servings: 4

Ingredients:

- 2 pounds beef stew meat, ground
- ½ pound white mushrooms, sliced
- 2 eggs, whisked
- 1 tablespoon olive oil
- 2 tablespoons parsley, chopped
- 2 garlic cloves, minced
- ½ cup coconut flour
- ½ cup mozzarella shredded
- A pinch of salt and black pepper

Directions:

In a bowl, combine the meat with the mushrooms and the other ingredients except the oil, and stir well. Transfer this into a loaf pan greased with the oil, bake in the oven at 375 degrees F for 50 minutes, cool down, slice and serve.

Nutrition: calories 264, fat 14, fiber 3, carbs 5, protein 24

Minty Beef
You need to make sure there's enough for everyone!

Preparation time: 10 minutes
Cooking time: 30 minutes
Servings: 4

Ingredients:

- 1 pound beef stew meat, cubed
- 2 tablespoons ghee, melted
- 2 shallots, chopped
- 1 cup beef stock
- ¼ cup mint, chopped
- ¼ cup parsley, chopped
- A pinch of salt and black pepper
- 2 garlic cloves, minced
- 2 tablespoons lime juice

Directions:

Heat up a pan with the ghee over medium heat, add the shallots, garlic and the meat and brown for 5 minutes. Add the rest of the ingredients, toss, bring to a simmer and cook over medium heat for 25 minutes more. Divide everything into bowls and serve.

Nutrition: calories 200, fat 4, fiber 1, carbs 3, protein 7

Parsley Pork and Beef Meatballs

A friendly meal can turn into a feast with this keto dish!

Preparation time: 10 minutes
Cooking time: 12 minutes
Servings: 4

Ingredients:

- 1 pound beef meat, ground
- ½ pound pork stew meat, ground
- 2 eggs, whisked
- ¼ cup coconut flour
- 1 cup parsley, minced
- 2 garlic cloves, minced
- 2 tablespoons ghee, melted
- A pinch of salt and black pepper

Directions:

In a bowl, combine the beef and pork meat with the other ingredients except the ghee, stir well and shape medium meatballs out of this mix. Heat up a pan with the ghee over medium heat, add the meatballs, cook them for 6 minutes on each side, divide between plates and serve.

Nutrition: calories 435, fat 23, fiber 4, carbs 6, protein 32

Beef with Kale and Leeks
This is so tasty!

Preparation time: 10 minutes
Cooking time: 30 minutes
Servings: 4

Ingredients:

- 2 tablespoons olive oil
- 1 pound beef stew meat, cubed
- 1 cup kale, torn
- 2 leeks, chopped
- 1 cup tomato passata
- A pinch of salt and black pepper
- 1 tablespoon cilantro, chopped
- 1 teaspoon sweet paprika
- ½ teaspoon rosemary, dried

Directions:

Heat up a pan with the oil over medium heat, add the leeks and the meat and brown for 5 minutes. Add the rest of the ingredients, bring to a simmer and cook over medium heat for 25 minutes more. Divide everything into bowls and serve.

Nutrition: calories 250, fat 5, fiber 1, carbs 3, protein 12

Sesame Beef
A friendly and casual meal requires such a keto dish!

Preparation time: 10 minutes
Cooking time: 35 minutes
Servings: 4

Ingredients:

- 2 pounds beef stew meat, cubed
- 2 tablespoons olive oil
- 2 garlic cloves, minced
- A pinch of salt and black pepper
- 1 tablespoon sesame seeds
- 1 cup mozzarella cheese, shredded
- ½ cup beef stock

Directions:

Heat up a pan with the oil over medium heat, add the meat and the garlic and brown for 5 minutes. Add the rest of the ingredients except the cheese, toss, bring to a simmer and cook for 25 minutes. Sprinkle the cheese on top, cook everything for 5 minutes more, divide between plates and serve.

Nutrition: calories 554, fat 51, fiber 3, carbs 5, protein 45

Marjoram Beef
It only takes a few minutes to make this special keto recipe!

Preparation time: 10 minutes
Cooking time: 30 minutes
Servings: 4

Ingredients:
- 1 pound beef stew meat, cubed
- 2 tablespoons ghee, melted
- 1 red onion, chopped
- 2 garlic cloves, minced
- 1 cup beef stock
- 2 teaspoons sweet paprika
- 1 tablespoon marjoram, chopped
- A pinch of salt and black pepper

Directions:
Heat up a pan with the ghee over medium heat, add the onion and the garlic and sauté for 5 minutes. Add the meat and brown for 5 minutes more. Add the rest of the ingredients, bring to a simmer and cook over medium heat for 20 minutes more. Divide everything into bowls and serve.

Nutrition: calories 320, fat 13, fiber 4, carbs 12, protein 40

Spiced Beef
This is really tasty! You must make it for your family tonight!

Preparation time: 10 minutes
Cooking time: 35 minutes
Servings: 4

Ingredients:
- 3 garlic cloves, minced
- 2 pounds beef stew meat, cubed
- ½ cup beef stock
- 2 tablespoons avocado oil
- 2 chilii peppers, chopped
- 1 teaspoon thyme, dried
- ½ teaspoon coriander, ground
- ½ teaspoon allspice, ground
- 2 teaspoons cumin, ground
- ½ teaspoon turmeric powder
- ¼ teaspoon nutmeg, ground
- A pinch of salt and black pepper
- 1 teaspoon garlic powder

Directions:
Heat up a pan with the oil over medium heat, add the garlic and the meat and brown for 5 minutes. Add the thyme, coriander and the rest of the ingredients, toss, bring to a simmer and cook over medium heat for 30 minutes more. Divide everything between plates and serve.

Nutrition: calories 267, fat 23, fiber 1, carbs 3, protein 12

Nutmeg Beef Bowls
This is a keto comfort food! Try it soon!

Preparation time: 10 minutes
Cooking time: 30 minutes
Servings: 4

Ingredients:

- 2 pounds beef stew meat, cubed
- 1 tablespoon ghee, melted
- 1 teaspoon nutmeg, ground
- 1 cup beef stock
- A pinch of salt and black pepper
- 2 tablespoons chives, chopped
- 1 cup tomato passata
- ¼ teaspoon garlic powder

Directions:

Heat up a pan with the ghee over medium heat, add the meat and brown for 5 minutes. Add the rest of the ingredients, bring to a simmer and cook over medium heat for 25 minutes more. Divide everything into bowls and serve.

Nutrition: calories 275, fat 7, fiber 2, carbs 4, protein 10

Pork and Eggplant Pan
These ingredients go perfectly together!

Preparation time: 10 minutes
Cooking time: 25 minutes
Servings: 4

Ingredients:

- 1 tablespoon olive oil
- 1 pound pork stew meat, cubed
- 1 cup eggplant, cubed
- A pinch of salt and black pepper
- 1 cup tomatoes, chopped
- 1 cup beef stock
- 2 tablespoons parsley, chopped

Directions:

Heat up a pan with the oil over medium heat, add the meat and brown for 5 minutes. Add the eggplant and the rest of the ingredients, cook everything over medium heat for 20 minutes more, divide into bowls and serve.

Nutrition: calories 200, fat 12, fiber 2, carbs 6, protein 15

Rosemary Lamb Chops
It's a perfect keto dish!

Preparation time: 10 minutes
Cooking time: 35 minutes
Servings: 4

Ingredients:
- 3 lamb chops
- A pinch of salt and black pepper
- 2 chili peppers, chopped
- 2 tablespoons olive oil
- 1 shallot, chopped
- Juice of 1 lime
- 1 cup beef stock
- ½ teaspoon rosemary, dried

Directions:
In a roasting pan, combine the lamb with the salt, pepper and the other ingredients, toss and bake at 390 degrees F for 35 minutes. Divide everything between plates and serve with a side salad.

Nutrition: calories 450, fat 34, fiber 2, carbs 6, protein 26

Cheesy Lamb Chops
It's a flavored dish you should try in the summer!

Preparation time: 10 minutes
Cooking time: 30 minutes
Servings: 4

Ingredients:
- 2 tablespoons olive oil
- 4 lamb chops
- Salt and black pepper to the taste
- 1 teaspoon cumin, ground
- 2 garlic cloves, minced
- 4 ounces cheddar, grated
- 1 cup mint, chopped

Directions:
In a roasting pan, combine the lamb chops with the other and the other ingredients except the cheese and rub well. Sprinkle the cheese on top, bake at 390 degrees F for 30 minutes, divide between plates and serve with a side salad.

Nutrition: calories 334, fat 33, fiber 3, carbs 5, protein 7

Moroccan Lamb
Try this Moroccan keto dish as soon as you can!

Preparation time: 10 minutes
Cooking time: 15 minutes
Servings: 4

Ingredients:
- 2 teaspoons paprika
- 2 garlic cloves, minced
- 2 teaspoons oregano, dried
- 2 tablespoons sumac
- 12 lamb cutlets
- ¼ cup olive oil
- 2 tablespoons water
- 2 teaspoons cumin, ground
- 4 carrots, sliced
- ¼ cup parsley, chopped
- 2 teaspoons harissa
- 1 tablespoon red wine vinegar
- Salt and black pepper to the taste
- 2 tablespoons black olives, pitted and sliced
- 6 radishes, thinly sliced

Directions:
In a bowl, mix cutlets with paprika, garlic, oregano, sumac, salt, pepper, half of the oil and the water and rub well. Put carrots in a pot, add water to cover, bring to a boil over medium high heat, cook for 2 minutes drain and put them in a salad bowl. Add olives and radishes over carrots. In another bowl, mix harissa with the rest of the oil, parsley, cumin, vinegar and a splash of water and stir well. Add this over carrots mix, season with salt and pepper and toss to coat. Heat up a kitchen grill over medium high heat, add lamb cutlets, grill them for 3 minutes on each side and divide them on plates. Add carrots salad on the side and serve.

Nutrition: calories 245, fat 32, fiber 6, carbs 4, protein 34

Delicious Lamb And Mustard Sauce

It's so rich and flavored and it's ready in only half an hour!

Preparation time: 10 minutes
Cooking time: 20 minutes
Servings: 4

Ingredients:

- 2 tablespoons olive oil
- 1 tablespoon fresh rosemary, chopped
- 2 garlic cloves, minced
- 1 and ½ pounds lamb chops
- Salt and black pepper to the taste
- 1 tablespoon shallot, chopped
- 2/3 cup heavy cream
- ½ cup beef stock
- 1 tablespoon mustard
- 2 teaspoons gluten free Worcestershire sauce
- 2 teaspoons lemon juice
- 1 teaspoon erythritol
- 2 tablespoons ghee
- A spring of rosemary
- A spring of thyme

Directions:

In a bowl, mix 1 tablespoon oil with garlic, salt, pepper and rosemary and whisk well. Add lamb chops, toss to coat and leave aside for a few minutes. Heat up a pan with the rest of the oil over medium high heat, add lamb chops, reduce heat to medium, cook them for 7 minutes, flip, cook them for 7 minutes more, transfer to a plate and keep them warm. Return pan to medium heat, add shallots, stir and cook for 3 minutes. Add stock, stir and cook for 1 minute. Add Worcestershire sauce, mustard, erythritol, cream, rosemary and thyme spring, stir and cook for 8 minutes. Add lemon juice, salt, pepper and the ghee, discard rosemary and thyme, stir well and take off heat. Divide lamb chops on plates, drizzle the sauce over them and serve.

Nutrition: calories 435, fat 30, fiber 4, carbs 5, protein 32

Tasty Lamb Curry

This lamb curry is going to surprise you for sure!

Preparation time: 10 minutes
Cooking time: 4 hours
Servings: 6

Ingredients:

- 2 tablespoons ginger, grated
- 2 garlic cloves, minced
- 2 teaspoons cardamom
- 1 red onion, chopped
- 6 cloves
- 1 pound lamb meat, cubed
- 2 teaspoons cumin powder
- 1 teaspoon garama masala
- ½ teaspoon chili powder
- 1 teaspoon turmeric
- 2 teaspoons coriander, ground
- 1 pound spinach
- 14 ounces canned tomatoes, chopped

Directions:

In your slow cooker, mix lamb with spinach, tomatoes, ginger, garlic, onion, cardamom, cloves, cumin, garam masala, chili, turmeric and coriander, stir, cover and cook on High for 4 hours. Uncover slow cooker, stir your chili, divide into bowls and serve.

Nutrition: calories 160, fat 6, fiber 3, carbs 7, protein 20

Tasty Lamb Stew

Don't bother looking for a Ketogenic dinner idea! This is the perfect one!

Preparation time: 10 minutes
Cooking time: 3 hours
Servings: 4

Ingredients:

- 1 yellow onion, chopped
- 3 carrots, chopped
- 2 pounds lamb, cubed
- 1 tomato, chopped
- 1 garlic clove, minced
- 2 tablespoons ghee
- 1 cup beef stock
- 1 cup white wine
- Salt and black pepper to the taste
- 2 rosemary springs
- 1 teaspoon thyme, chopped

Directions:

Heat up a Dutch oven over medium high heat, add oil and heat up. Add lamb, salt and pepper, brown on all sides and transfer to a plate. Add onion to the pot and cook for 2 minutes. Add carrots, tomato, garlic, ghee, stick, wine, salt, pepper, rosemary and thyme, stir and cook for a couple of minutes. Return lamb to pot, stir, reduce heat to medium low, cover and cook for 4 hours. Discard rosemary springs, add more salt and pepper, stir, divide into bowls and serve.

Nutrition: calories 700, fat 43, fiber 6, carbs 10, protein 67

Delicious Lamb Casserole

Serve this keto dish on a Sunday!

Preparation time: 10 minutes
Cooking time: 1 hour and 40 minutes
Servings: 2
Ingredients:

- 2 garlic cloves, minced
- 1 red onion, chopped
- 1 tablespoon olive oil
- 1 celery stick, chopped
- 10 ounces lamb fillet, cut in medium pieces
- Salt and black pepper to the taste
- 1 and ¼ cups lamb stock
- 2 carrots, chopped
- ½ tablespoon rosemary, chopped
- 1 leek, chopped
- 1 tablespoon mint sauce
- 1 teaspoon stevia
- 1 tablespoon tomato puree
- ½ cauliflower, florets separated
- ½ celeriac, chopped
- 2 tablespoons ghee

Directions:

Heat up a pot with the oil over medium heat, add garlic, onion and celery, stir and cook for 5 minutes. Add lamb pieces, stir and cook for 3 minutes. Add carrot, leek, rosemary, stock, tomato puree, mint sauce and stevia, stir, bring to a boil, cover and cook for 1 hour and 30 minutes. Heat up a pot with water over medium heat, add celeriac, cover and simmer for 10 minutes. Add cauliflower florets, cook for 15 minutes, drain everything and mix with salt, pepper and ghee. Mash using a potato masher and divide mash on plates. Add lamb and veggies mix on top and serve.

Nutrition: calories 324, fat 4, fiber 5, carbs 8, protein 20

Amazing Lamb

This is a keto slow cooked lamb you will love for sure!

Preparation time: 10 minutes
Cooking time: 8 hours
Servings: 6
Ingredients:

- 2 pounds lamb leg
- Salt and black pepper to the taste
- 1 tablespoon maple extract
- 2 tablespoons mustard
- ¼ cup olive oil
- 4 thyme spring
- 6 mint leaves
- 1 teaspoon garlic, minced
- A pinch of rosemary, dried

Directions:

Put the oil in your slow cooker. Add lamb, salt, pepper, maple extract, mustard, rosemary and garlic, rub well, cover and cook on Low for 7 hours. Add mint and thyme and cook for 1 more hour. Leave lamb to cool down a bit before slicing and serving with pan juices on top.

Nutrition: calories 400, fat 34, fiber 1, carbs 3, protein 26

Lavender Lamb Chops

It's amazing and very flavored! Try it as son as you can!

Preparation time: 10 minutes
Cooking time: 25 minutes
Servings: 4

Ingredients:

- 2 tablespoons rosemary, chopped
- 1 and ½ pounds lamb chops
- Salt and black pepper to the taste
- 1 tablespoon lavender, chopped
- 2 garlic cloves, minced
- 3 red oranges, cut in halves
- 2 small pieces of orange peel
- A drizzle of olive oil
- 1 teaspoon ghee

Directions:

In a bowl, mix lamb chops with salt, pepper, rosemary, lavender, garlic and orange peel, toss to coat and leave aside for a couple of hours. Grease your kitchen grill with ghee, heat up over medium high heat, place lamb chops on it, cook for 3 minutes, flip, squeeze 1 orange half over them, cook for 3 minutes more, flip them again, cook them for 2 minutes and squeeze another orange half over them. Place lamb chops on a plate and keep them warm for now. Add remaining orange halves on preheated grill, cook them for 3 minutes, flip and cook them for another 3 minutes. Divide lamb chops on plates, add orange halves on the side, drizzle some olive oil over them and serve.

Nutrition: calories 250, fat 5, fiber 1, carbs 5, protein 8

Crusted Lamb Chops

This is easy to make and it will taste very good!

Preparation time: 10 minutes
Cooking time: 15 minutes
Servings: 4

Ingredients:

- 2 lamb racks, cut into chops
- Salt and black pepper to the taste
- 3 tablespoons paprika
- ¾ cup cumin powder
- 1 teaspoon chili powder

Directions:

In a bowl, mix paprika with cumin, chili, salt and pepper and stir. Add lamb chops and rub them well. Heat up your grill over medium temperature, add lamb chops, cook for 5 minutes, flip and cook for 5 minutes more. Flip them again, cook for 2 minutes and then for 2 minutes more on the other side again.

Nutrition: calories 200, fat 5, fiber 2, carbs 4, protein 8

Lamb And Orange Dressing
You will love this dish!

Preparation time: 10 minutes
Cooking time: 4 hours
Servings: 4

Ingredients:

- 2 lamb shanks
- Salt and black pepper to the taste
- 1 garlic head, peeled
- 4 tablespoons olive oil
- Juice from ½ lemon
- Zest from ½ lemon
- ½ teaspoon oregano, dried

Directions:

In your slow cooker, mix lamb with salt and pepper. Add garlic, cover and cook on High for 4 hours. Meanwhile, in a bowl, mix lemon juice with lemon zest, some salt and pepper, the olive oil and oregano and whisk very well. Uncover your slow cooker, shred lamb meat and discard bone and divide on plates. Drizzle the lemon dressing all over and serve.

Nutrition: calories 160, fat 7, fiber 3, carbs 5, protein 12

Lamb Riblets And Tasty Mint Pesto
The pesto makes this keto dish really surprising and tasty!

Preparation time: 1 hour
Cooking time: 2 hours
Servings: 4

Ingredients:

- 1 cup parsley
- 1 cup mint
- 1 small yellow onion, roughly chopped
- 1/3 cup pistachios
- 1 teaspoon lemon zest
- 5 tablespoons avocado oil
- Salt to the taste
- 2 pounds lamb riblets
- ½ onion, chopped
- 5 garlic cloves, minced
- Juice from 1 orange

Directions:

In your food processor, mix parsley with mint, 1 small onion, pistachios, lemon zest, salt and avocado oil and blend very well. Rub lamb with this mix, place in a bowl, cover and leave in the fridge for 1 hour. Transfer lamb to a baking dish, add garlic and ½ onion to the dish as well, drizzle orange juice and bake in the oven at 250 degrees F for 2 hours. Divide on plates and serve.

Nutrition: calories 200, fat 4, fiber 1, carbs 5, protein 7

Lamb With Fennel And Figs
It will have a divine taste!

Preparation time: 10 minutes
Cooking time: 40 minutes
Servings: 4

Ingredients:

- 12 ounces lamb racks
- 2 fennel bulbs, sliced
- Salt and black pepper to the taste
- 2 tablespoons olive oil
- 4 figs, cut in halves
- 1/8 cup apple cider vinegar
- 1 tablespoon swerve

Directions:

In a bowl, mix fennel with figs, vinegar, swerve and oil, toss to coat well and transfer to a baking dish. Season with salt and pepper, introduce in the oven at 400 degrees F and bake for 15 minutes. Season lamb with salt and pepper, place into a heated pan over medium high heat and cook for a couple of minutes. Add lamb to the baking dish with the fennel and figs, introduce in the oven and bake for 20 minutes more. Divide everything on plates and serve.

Nutrition: calories 230, fat 3, fiber 3, carbs 5, protein 10

Baked Veal And Cabbage
Everyone should learn how to make this wonderful dish!

Preparation time: 10 minutes
Cooking time: 40 minutes
Servings: 4

Ingredients:

- 17 ounces veal, cut into cubes
- 1 cabbage, shredded
- Salt and black pepper to the taste
- 3.4 ounces ham, roughly chopped
- 1 small yellow onion, chopped
- 2 garlic cloves, minced
- 1 tablespoon ghee
- ½ cup parmesan, grated
- ½ cup sour cream

Directions:

Heat up a pot with the ghee over medium high heat, add onion, stir and cook for 2 minutes. Add garlic, stir and cook for 1 minute more. Add ham and veal, stir and cook until they brown a bit. Add cabbage, stir and cook until it softens and the meat is tender. Add cream, salt, pepper and cheese, stir gently, introduce in the oven at 350 degrees F and bake for 20 minutes. Divide on plates and serve.

Nutrition: calories 230, fat 7, fiber 4, carbs 6, protein 29

Delicious Beef Bourguignon

It might sound a bit fancy, but it's really easy to make!

Preparation time: 3 hours and 10 minutes
Cooking time: 5 hours and 15 minutes
Servings: 8

Ingredients:
- 3 tablespoons olive oil
- 2 tablespoons onion, chopped
- 1 tablespoon parsley flakes
- 1 and ½ cups red wine
- 1 teaspoon thyme, dried
- Salt and black pepper to the taste
- 1 bay leaf
- 1/3 cup almond flour
- 4 pounds beef, cubed
- 24 small white onions
- 8 bacon slices, chopped
- 2 garlic cloves, minced
- 1 pound mushrooms, roughly chopped

Directions:

In a bowl, mix wine with olive oil, minced onion, thyme, parsley, salt, pepper and bay leaf and whisk well. Add beef cubes, stir and leave aside for 3 hours.

Drain meat and reserve 1 cup of marinade. Add flour over meat and toss to coat. Heat up a pan over medium high heat, add bacon, stir and cook until it browns a bit. Add onions, stir and cook for 3 minutes more. Add garlic, stir, cook for 1 minute and transfer everything to a slow cooker. Also add meat to the slow cooker and stir. Heat up the pan with the bacon fat over medium high heat, add mushrooms and white onions, stir and sauté them for a couple of minutes. Add these to slow cooker as well, also add reserved marinade, some salt and pepper, cover and cook on High for 5 hours. Divide on plates and serve.

Nutrition: calories 435, fat 16, fiber 1, carbs 7, protein 45

Roasted Beef

It's as simple as that!

Preparation time: 10 minutes
Cooking time: 8 hours
Servings: 8

Ingredients:

- 5 pounds beef roast
- Salt and black pepper to the taste
- ½ teaspoon celery salt
- 2 teaspoons chili powder
- 1 tablespoon avocado oil
- 1 tablespoon sweet paprika
- A pinch of cayenne pepper
- ½ teaspoon garlic powder
- ½ cup beef stock
- 1 tablespoon garlic, minced
- ¼ teaspoon dry mustard

Directions:

Heat up a pan with the oil over medium high heat, add beef roast and brown it on all sides. In a bowl, mix paprika with chili powder, celery salt, salt, pepper, cayenne, garlic powder and mustard powder and stir. Add roast, rub well and transfer it to a Crockpot. Add beef stock and garlic over roast and cook on Low for 8 hours. Transfer beef to a cutting board, leave it to cool down a bit, slice and divide on plates. Strain juices from the pot, drizzle over meat and serve.

Nutrition: calories 180, fat 5, fiber 1, carbs 5, protein 25

Amazing Beef Stew

You should try this Ketogenic stew today!

Preparation time: 10 minutes
Cooking time: 4 hours and 10 minutes
Servings: 4

Ingredients:

- 8 ounces pancetta, chopped
- 4 pounds beef, cubed
- 4 garlic cloves, minced
- 2 brown onions, chopped
- 2 tablespoons olive oil
- 4 tablespoons red vinegar
- 4 cups beef stock
- 2 tablespoons tomato paste
- 2 cinnamon sticks
- 3 lemon peel strips
- A handful parsley, chopped
- 4 thyme springs
- 2 tablespoons ghee
- Salt and black pepper to the taste

Directions:

Heat up a pan with the oil over medium high heat, add pancetta, onion and garlic, stir and cook fro 5 minutes. Add beef, stir and cook until it browns. Add vinegar, salt, pepper, stock, tomato paste, cinnamon, lemon peel, thyme and ghee, stir, cook for 3 minutes and transfer everything to your slow cooker. Cover and cook on High for 4 hours. Discard cinnamon, lemon peel and thyme, add parsley, stir and divide into bowls. Serve hot.

Nutrition: calories 250, fat 6, fiber 1, carbs 7, protein 33

Delicious Pork Stew

A wonderful keto stew is all you need today!

Preparation time: 10 minutes
Cooking time: 1 hour and 20 minutes
Servings: 12

Ingredients:

2 tablespoons coconut oil
4 pounds pork, cubed
Salt and black pepper to the taste
2 tablespoons ghee
3 garlic cloves, minced
¾ cup beef stock
¾ cup apple cider vinegar
3 carrots, chopped
1 cabbage head, shredded
½ cup green onion, chopped
1 cup whipping cream

Directions:

Heat up a pan with the ghee and the oil over medium high heat, add pork and brown it for a few minutes on each side. Add vinegar and stock, stir well and bring to a simmer. Add cabbage, garlic, salt and pepper, stir, cover and cook for 1 hour. Add carrots and green onions, stir and cook for 15 minutes more. Add whipping cream, stir for 1 minute, divide on plates and serve.

Nutrition: calories 400, fat 25, fiber 3, carbs 6, protein 43

Delicious Sausage Stew

We recommend you to try this stew if you are on a keto diet!

Preparation time: 10 minutes
Cooking time: 20 minutes
Servings: 9

Ingredients:

- 1 pound smoked sausage, sliced
- 1 green bell pepper, chopped
- 2 yellow onions, chopped
- Salt and black pepper to the taste
- 1 cup parsley, chopped
- 8 green onions, chopped
- ¼ cup avocado oil
- 1 cup beef stock
- 6 garlic cloves
- 28 ounces canned tomatoes, chopped
- 16 ounces okra, chopped
- 8 ounces tomato sauce
- 2 tablespoons coconut aminos
- 1 tablespoon gluten free hot sauce

Directions:

Heat up a pot with the oil over medium high heat, add sausages, stir and cook for 2 minutes. Add onion, bell pepper, green onions, parsley, salt and pepper, stir and cook for 2 minutes more. Add stock, garlic, tomatoes, okra, tomato sauce, coconut aminos and hot sauce, stir, bring to a simmer and cook for 15 minutes. Add more salt and pepper, stir, divide into bowls and serve.

Nutrition: calories 274, fat 20, fiber 4, carbs 7, protein 10

Burgundy Beef Stew

It's time to learn how to make a special keto stew for your loved ones!

Preparation time: 10 minutes
Cooking time: 3 hours
Servings: 7
Ingredients:

- 2 pounds beef chuck roast, cubed
- 15 ounces canned tomatoes, chopped
- 4 carrots, chopped
- Salt and black pepper to the taste
- ½ pounds mushrooms, sliced
- 2 celery ribs, chopped
- 2 yellow onions, chopped
- 1 cup beef stock
- 1 tablespoon thyme, chopped
- ½ teaspoon mustard powder
- 3 tablespoons almond flour
- 1 cup water

Directions:

Heat up an oven proof pot over medium high heat, add beef cubes, stir and brown them for a couple of minutes on each side. Add tomatoes, mushrooms, onions, carrots, celery, salt, pepper mustard, stock and thyme and stir. In a bowl mix water with flour and stir well. Add this to the pot, stir well, introduce in the oven and bake at 325 degrees F for 3 hours. Stir every half an hour. Divide into bowls and serve.

Nutrition: calories 275, fat 13, fiber 4, carbs 7, protein 28

Cuban Beef Stew

A Cuban keto stew can make your day a lot better!

Preparation time: 10 minutes
Cooking time: 6 hours
Servings: 8
Ingredients:

- 2 yellow onions, chopped
- 2 tablespoons avocado oil
- 2 pounds beef roast, cubed
- 2 green bell peppers, chopped
- 1 habanero pepper, chopped
- 4 jalapenos, chopped
- 14 ounces canned tomatoes, chopped
- 2 tablespoons cilantro, chopped
- 6 garlic cloves, minced
- ½ cup water
- Salt and black pepper to the taste
- 1 and ½ teaspoons cumin, ground
- 4 teaspoons bouillon granules
- ½ cup black olives, pitted and chopped
- 1 teaspoon oregano, dried

Directions:

Heat up a pan with the oil over medium high heat, add beef, brown it on all sides and transfer to a slow cooker. Add green bell peppers, onions, jalapenos, habanero pepper, tomatoes, garlic, water, bouillon, cilantro, oregano, cumin, salt and pepper and stir. Cover slow cooker and cook on Low for 6 hours. Add olives, stir, divide into bowls and serve.

Nutrition: calories 305, fat 14, fiber 4, carbs 8, protein 25

Ham Stew
It's perfect for dinner tonight!

Preparation time: 10 minutes
Cooking time: 4 hours
Servings: 6

Ingredients:

- 8 ounces cheddar cheese, grated
- 14 ounces chicken stock
- ½ teaspoon garlic powder
- ½ teaspoon onion powder
- Salt and black pepper to the taste
- 4 garlic cloves, minced
- ¼ cup heavy cream
- 3 cups ham, chopped
- 16 ounces cauliflower florets

Directions:

In your Crockpot, mix ham with stock, cheese, cauliflower, garlic powder, onion powder, salt, pepper, garlic and heavy cream, stir, cover and cook on High for 4 hours. Stir, divide into bowls and serve.

Nutrition: calories 320, fat 20, fiber 3, carbs 6, protein 23

Delicious Veal Stew
No matter how busy you are, you can make the time to prepare this keto dish!

Preparation time: 10 minutes
Cooking time: 2 hours and 10 minutes
Servings: 12

Ingredients:

- 2 tablespoons avocado oil
- 3 pounds veal, cubed
- 1 yellow onion, chopped
- 1 small garlic clove, minced
- Salt and black pepper to the taste
- 1 cup water
- 1 and ½ cups marsala wine
- 10 ounces canned tomato paste
- 1 carrot, chopped
- 7 ounces mushrooms, chopped
- 3 egg yolks
- ½ cup heavy cream
- 2 teaspoons oregano, dried

Directions:

Heat up a pot with the oil over medium high heat, add veal, stir and brown it for a few minutes. Add garlic and onion, stir and cook for 2-3 minutes more. Add wine, water, oregano, tomato paste, mushrooms, carrots, salt and pepper, stir, bring to a boil, cover, reduce heat to low and cook for 1 hour and 45 minutes. In a bowl, mix cream with egg yolks and whisk well. Pour this into the pot, stir, cook for 15 minutes more, add more salt and pepper if needed, divide into bowls and serve.

Nutrition: calories 254, fat 15, fiber 1, carbs 3, protein 23

Veal And Tomatoes Dish

Make a special dinner for your loved ones! Try this keto recipe!

Preparation time: 10 minutes
Cooking time: 40 minutes
Servings: 4

Ingredients:

- 4 medium veal leg steaks
- A drizzle of avocado oil
- 2 garlic cloves, minced
- 1 red onion, chopped
- Salt and black pepper to the taste
- 2 teaspoons sage, chopped
- 15 ounces canned tomatoes, chopped
- 2 tablespoons parsley, chopped
- 1 ounce bocconcini, sliced
- Green beans, steamed for serving

Directions:

Heat up a pan with the oil over medium high heat, add veal, cook for 2 minutes on each side and transfer to a baking dish. Return pan to heat, add onion, stir and cook for 4 minutes. Add sage and garlic, stir and cook for 1 minute. Add tomatoes, stir, bring to a boil and cook for 10 minutes. Pour this over veal, add bocconcini and parsley, introduce in the oven at 350 degrees G and bake for 20 minutes. Divide on plates and serve with steamed green beans on the side.

Nutrition: calories 276, fat 6, fiber 4, carbs 5, protein 36

Veal Parmesan

It's a very popular keto dish and you should learn how to make it!

Preparation time: 10 minutes
Cooking time: 1 hour and 10 minutes
Servings: 6

Ingredients:

- 8 veal cutlets
- 2/3 cup parmesan, grated
- 8 provolone cheese slices
- Salt and black pepper to the taste
- 5 cups tomato sauce
- A pinch of garlic salt
- Cooking spray
- 2 tablespoons ghee
- 2 tablespoons coconut oil, melted
- 1 teaspoon Italian seasoning

Directions:

Season veal cutlets with salt, pepper and garlic salt and drub. Heat up a pan with the ghee and the oil over medium high heat, add veal and cook until they brown on all sides. Spread half of the tomato sauce on the bottom of a baking dish which you've greased with some cooking spray. Add veal cutlets, then sprinkle Italian seasoning and spread the rest of the sauce. Cover dish, introduce in the oven at 350 degrees F and bake for 40 minutes. Uncover dish, spread provolone cheese and sprinkle parmesan, introduce in the oven again and bake for 15 minutes more. Divide on plates and serve.

Nutrition: calories 362, fat 21, fiber 2, carbs 6, protein 26

Veal Piccata
Make this for your loved one tonight!

Preparation time: 10 minutes
Cooking time: 15 minutes
Servings: 2

Ingredients:
- 2 tablespoons ghee
- ¼ cup white wine
- ¼ cup chicken stock
- 1 and ½ tablespoons capers
- 1 garlic clove, minced
- 8 ounces veal scallops
- Salt and black pepper to the taste

Directions:
Heat up a pan with half of the butter over medium high heat, add veal cutlets, season with salt and pepper, cook for 1 minute on each side and transfer to a plate. Heat up the pan again over medium heat, add garlic, stir and cook for 1 minute. Add wine, stir and simmer for 2 minutes. Add stock, capers, salt, pepper, the rest of the ghee and return veal to pan. Stir everything, cover pan and cook piccata on medium low heat until veal is tender.

Nutrition: calories 204, fat 12, fiber 1, carbs 5, protein 10

Delicious Roasted Sausage
It's very easy to make at home tonight!

Preparation time: 10 minutes
Cooking time: 1 hour
Servings: 6

Ingredients:
- 3 red bell peppers, chopped
- 2 pounds Italian pork sausage, sliced
- Salt and black pepper to the taste
- 2 pounds Portobello mushrooms, sliced
- 2 sweet onions, chopped
- 1 tablespoon swerve
- A drizzle of olive oil

Directions:
In a baking dish, mix sausage slices with oil, salt, pepper, bell pepper, mushrooms, onion and swerve. Toss to coat, introduce in the oven at 300 degrees F and bake for 1 hour. Divide on plates and serve hot.

Nutrition: calories 130, fat 12, fiber 1, carbs 3, protein 9

Baked Sausage And Kale
This keto dish will be ready in 20 minutes!

Preparation time: 5 minutes
Cooking time: 30 minutes
Servings: 4

Ingredients:
- 1 cup yellow onion, chopped
- 1 and ½ pound Italian pork sausage, sliced
- ½ cup red bell pepper, chopped
- Salt and black pepper to the taste
- 5 pounds kale, chopped
- 1 teaspoon garlic, minced
- ¼ cup red hot chili pepper, chopped
- 1 cup water

Directions:
Heat up a pan over medium high heat, add sausage, stir, reduce heat to medium and cook for 10 minutes. Add onions, stir and cook for 3-4 minutes more. Add bell pepper and garlic, stir and cook for 1 minute. Add kale, chili pepper, salt, pepper and water, stir and cook for 10 minutes more. Divide on plates and serve.

Nutrition: calories 150, fat 4, fiber 1, carbs 2, protein 12

Sausage With Tomatoes And Cheese
It's a surprising and very tasty combination!

Preparation time: 10 minutes
Cooking time: 30 minutes
Servings: 4

Ingredients:
- 2 ounces coconut oil, melted
- 2 pounds Italian pork sausage, chopped
- 1 onion, sliced
- 4 sun dried tomatoes, thinly sliced
- Salt and black pepper to the taste
- ½ pound gouda cheese, grated
- 3 yellow bell peppers, chopped
- 3 orange bell peppers, chopped
- A pinch of red pepper flakes
- A handful parsley, thinly sliced

Directions:
Heat up a pan with the oil over medium high heat, add sausage slices, stir, cook for 3 minutes on each side, transfer to a plate and leave aside for now. Heat up the pan again over medium heat, add onion, yellow and orange bell peppers and tomatoes, stir and cook for 5 minutes. Add pepper flakes, salt and pepper, stir well, cook for 1 minute and take off heat. Arrange sausage slices into a baking dish, add bell peppers mix on top, add parsley and gouda as well, introduce in the oven at 350 degrees F and bake for 15 minutes. Divide on plates and serve hot.

Nutrition: calories 200, fat 5, fiber 3, carbs 6, protein 14

Delicious Sausage Salad
Check this out! It's very tasty!

Preparation time: 10 minutes
Cooking time: 7 minutes
Servings: 4

Ingredients:
- 8 pork sausage links, sliced
- 1 pound mixed cherry tomatoes, cut in halves
- 4 cups baby spinach
- 1 tablespoon avocado oil
- 1 pound mozzarella cheese, cubed
- 2 tablespoons lemon juice
- 2/3 cup basil pesto
- Salt and black pepper to the taste

Directions:
Heat up a pan with the oil over medium high heat, add sausage slices, stir and cook them for 4 minutes on each side. Meanwhile, in a salad bowl, mix spinach with mozzarella, tomatoes, salt, pepper, lemon juice and pesto and toss to coat.
Add sausage pieces, toss again and serve.

Nutrition: calories 250, fat 12, fiber 3, carbs 8, protein 18

Delicious Sausage And Peppers Soup
This keto soup will hypnotize everyone!

Preparation time: 10 minutes
Cooking time: 1 hour and 10 minutes
Servings: 6

Ingredients:
- 1 tablespoon avocado oil
- 32 ounces pork sausage meat
- 10 ounces canned tomatoes and jalapenos, chopped
- 10 ounces spinach
- 1 green bell pepper, chopped
- 4 cups beef stock
- 1 teaspoon onion powder
- Salt and black pepper to the taste
- 1 tablespoon cumin
- 1 tablespoon chili powder
- 1 teaspoon garlic powder
- 1 teaspoon Italian seasoning

Directions:
Heat up a pot with the oil over medium heat, add sausage, stir and brown for a couple of minutes on all sides. Add green bell pepper, salt and pepper, stir and cook for 3 minutes. Add tomatoes and jalapenos, stir and cook for 2 minutes more. Add spinach, stir, cover and cook for 7 minutes. Add stock, onion powder, garlic powder, chili powder, cumin, salt, pepper and Italian seasoning, stir everything, cover pot and cook for 30 minutes. Uncover pot and cook soup for 15 minutes more. Divide into bowls and serve.

Nutrition: calories 524, fat 43, fiber 2, carbs 4, protein 26

Italian Sausage Soup

Everyone can make this amazing keto soup! It's so tasty and healthy!

Preparation time: 10 minutes
Cooking time: 30 minutes
Servings: 12

Ingredients:

- 64 ounces chicken stock
- A drizzle of avocado oil
- 1 cup heavy cream
- 10 ounces spinach
- 6 bacon slices, chopped
- 1 pound radishes, chopped
- 2 garlic cloves, minced
- Salt and black pepper to the taste
- A pinch of red pepper flakes, crushed
- 1 yellow onion, chopped
- 1 and ½ pounds hot pork sausage, chopped

Directions:

Heat up a pot with a drizzle of avocado oil over medium high heat, add sausage, onion and garlic, stir and brown for a few minutes. Add stock, spinach and radishes, stir and bring to a simmer. Add bacon, cream, salt, pepper and red pepper flakes, stir and cook for 20 minutes more. Divide into bowls and serve.

Nutrition: calories 291, fat 22, fiber 2, carbs 4, protein 17

Ketogenic Vegetable Recipes

Broccoli Cream
This is so textured and delicious!

Preparation time: 10 minutes
Cooking time: 20 minutes
Servings: 4

Ingredients:
- 1 pound broccoli florets
- 4 cups vegetable stock
- 2 shallots, chopped
- 1 teaspoon chili powder
- A pinch of salt and black pepper
- 2 garlic cloves, minced
- 2 tablespoons olive oil, chopped
- 1 tablespoon dill, chopped

Directions:
Heat up a pot with the oil over medium high heat, add the shallots and the garlic and sauté for 2 minutes. Add the broccoli and the other ingredients, bring to a simmer and cook over medium heat for 18 minutes. Blend the mix using an immersion blender, divide the cream into bowls and serve.

Nutrition: calories 111, fat 8, fiber 3.3, carbs 10.2, protein 3.7

Cauliflower and Tomatoes Mix
This veggie mix is just delicious!

Preparation time: 10 minutes
Cooking time: 30 minutes
Servings: 4

Ingredients:
- 1 pound cauliflower florets
- ½ pound cherry tomatoes, halved
- 2 tablespoons avocado oil
- 2 shallots, chopped
- 2 garlic cloves, minced
- A pinch of salt and black pepper
- 1 cup vegetable stock
- 1 tablespoon coriander, chopped
- ½ teaspoon allspice, ground

Directions:
Heat up a pan with the oil over medium heat, add the shallots and the garlic and sauté for 2 minutes. Add the cauliflower and the other ingredients, toss, bring to a simmer and cook over medium heat for 28 minutes more. Divide everything between plates and serve.

Nutrition: calories 57, fat 1.7, fiber 3.9, carbs 10.7, protein 3.1

Shallots and Kale Soup
A keto soup sounds pretty amazing, doesn't it?

Preparation time: 10 minutes
Cooking time: 20 minutes
Servings: 4

Ingredients:

- 4 cups chicken stock
- 1 pound kale, torn
- 2 shallots, chopped
- A pinch of salt and black pepper
- 1 tablespoon olive oil
- 2 teaspoons coconut aminos
- 1 tablespoon cilantro, chopped

Directions:
Heat up a pot with the oil over medium heat, add the shallots and sauté for 5 minutes. Add the kale, stock and the other ingredients, bring to a simmer and cook over medium heat for 15 minutes more. Divide the soup into bowls and serve.

Nutrition: calories 98, fat 4.1, fiber 1.7, carbs 13.1, protein 4.1

Hot Kale Pan
You can even have this for dinner!

Preparation time: 10 minutes
Cooking time: 23 minutes
Servings: 4

Ingredients:

- 1 red onion, chopped
- 1 pound kale, roughly torn
- 1 cup baby bella mushrooms, halved
- A pinch of salt and black pepper
- 1 tablespoon olive oil
- 3 garlic cloves, minced
- ½ teaspoon hot paprika
- ½ tablespoon red pepper flakes, crushed
- 1 tablespoon dill, chopped
- 3 tablespoons coconut aminos

Directions:
Heat up a pan with the oil over medium heat, add the onion and the garlic and sauté for 5 minutes. Add the mushrooms, and sauté them for 3 minutes more.
Add the kale and the other ingredients, toss, cook over medium heat for 15 minutes more, divide into bowls and serve.

Nutrition: calories 100, fat 3, fiber 1, carbs 2, protein 6

Baked Broccoli

It's simple, it's easy and very delicious!

Preparation time: 10 minutes
Cooking time: 20 minutes
Servings: 4

Ingredients:

- 2 garlic cloves, minced
- 2 tablespoons olive oil
- 1 pound broccoli florets
- ½ teaspoon nutmeg, ground
- ½ teaspoons rosemary, dried
- A pinch of salt and black pepper

Directions:

In a roasting pan, combine the broccoli with the garlic and the other ingredients, toss and bake at 400 degrees F for 20 minutes. Divide the mix between plates and serve.

Nutrition: calories 150, fat 4.1, fiber 1, carbs 3.2, protein 2

Leeks Cream

This will impress you!

Preparation time: 10 minutes
Cooking time: 30 minutes
Servings: 4

Ingredients:

- 4 leeks, sliced
- 4 cups vegetable stock
- 1 tablespoon olive oil
- 2 shallots, chopped
- 1 tablespoon rosemary, chopped
- A pinch of salt and black pepper
- 1 cup heavy cream
- 1 tablespoon chives, chopped

Directions:

Heat up a pot with the oil over medium high heat, add the shallots and the leeks and sauté for 5 minutes. Add the stock and the other ingredients except the chives, bring to a simmer and cook over medium heat for 25 minutes stirring from time to time. Blend the soup using an immersion blender, ladle it into bowls, sprinkle the chives on top and serve.

Nutrition: calories 150, fat 3, fiber 1, carbs 2, protein 6

Fennel Soup
It's so delightful and delicious! Try it!

Preparation time: 10 minutes
Cooking time: 25 minutes
Servings: 4

Ingredients:
- 2 fennel bulb, sliced
- 2 tablespoons olive oil
- 2 shallots, chopped
- 3 garlic cloves, minced
- 4 cups chicken stock
- A pinch of salt and black pepper
- 1 cup heavy cream
- 1 tablespoon dill, chopped

Directions:
Heat up a pot with the oil over medium heat, add the shallots and the garlic and sauté for 5 minutes. Add the fennel and the other ingredients, bring to a simmer, cook over medium heat for 20 minutes more, blend using an immersion blender, divide into bowls and serve.

Nutrition: calories 140, fat 2, fiber 1, carbs 5, protein 10

Cauliflower and Green Beans
This Iranian style keto stew is so tasty and easy to make!

Preparation time: 10 minutes
Cooking time: 30 minutes
Servings: 4

Ingredients:
- 1 pound cauliflower florets
- 1 red onion, chopped
- 1 tablespoon olive oil
- 2 garlic cloves minced
- 1 cup tomato passata
- A pinch of salt and black pepper
- ½ pound green beans, trimmed and halved
- 1 tablespoon cilantro, chopped

Directions:
Heat up a pot with the oil over medium high heat, add the onion and the garlic and sauté for 5 minutes. Add the cauliflower and the other ingredients, toss and cook everything for 25 minutes more. Divide everything between plates and serve.

Nutrition: calories 93, fat 3.7, fiber 5.9, carbs 13.7, protein 4.1

Bok Choy Soup

It's a textured and creamy keto mix you have to try soon!

Preparation time: 10 minutes
Cooking time: 25 minutes
Servings: 4

Ingredients:

- 2 tablespoons coconut oil, melted
- 1 pound bok choy, torn
- 2 shallots, chopped
- 4 cups chicken stock
- 1 cup heavy cream
- 1 tablespoon cilantro, chopped
- A pinch of salt and black pepper
- ½ teaspoon nutmeg, ground

Directions:

Heat up a pot with the oil over medium heat, add the shallots and sauté for 5 minutes. Add the bok choy and the other ingredients, bring to a simmer and cook over medium heat for 20 minutes. Blend the soup using an immersion blender, divide into bowls and serve.

Nutrition: calories 192, fat 18.8, fiber 1.2, carbs 5.1, protein 3.2

Cabbage Sauté

This is so tasty!

Preparation time: 10 minutes
Cooking time: 20 minutes
Servings: 4

Ingredients:

- 2 garlic cloves, minced
- 2 shallots, chopped
- 1 tablespoon olive oil
- 1 green cabbage head, shredded
- 1 cup tomatoes, cubed
- 1 teaspoon lime juice
- A pinch of salt and black pepper
- 1 tablespoon cilantro, chopped

Directions:

Heat up a pan with the oil over medium high heat, add the shallots and the garlic and sauté for 5 minutes. Add the cabbage and the other ingredients, toss and cook over medium heat for 15 minutes more. Divide everything between plates and serve.

Nutrition: calories 89, fat 3.8, fiber 5.1, carbs 13.5, protein 2.9

Mustard Greens Sauté
This tasty dish will be ready in not time!

Preparation time: 10 minutes
Cooking time: 20 minutes
Servings: 4

Ingredients:
- 1 tablespoon olive oil
- 1 pound mustard greens, roughly chopped
- 2 garlic cloves, minced
- 2 spring onions, chopped
- A pinch of salt and black pepper
- ½ cup chicken stock
- 1 tablespoon balsamic vinegar
- 1 tablespoon cilantro, chopped

Directions:
Heat up a pan with the oil over medium heat, add the garlic and the spring onions, stir and sauté for 5 minutes. Add the mustard greens and the other ingredients, bring to a simmer and cook over medium heat for 15 minutes more. Divide everything between plates and serve.

Nutrition: calories 150, fat 12, fiber 2, carbs 4, protein 8

Bok Choy and Tomatoes
This is just fantastic!

Preparation time: 10 minutes
Cooking time: 20 minutes
Servings: 4

Ingredients:
- 1 pound bok choy
- 2 shallots, chopped
- 1 tablespoon olive oil
- 2 cups tomatoes, cubed
- 1 tablespoon balsamic vinegar
- ½ cup vegetable stock
- A pinch of salt and black pepper
- 1 teaspoon rosemary, dried
- 1 teaspoon fennel powder
- 1 tablespoon chives, chopped

Directions:
Heat up a pan with the oil over medium heat, add the shallots and sauté for 3 minutes. Add the bok choy and the other ingredients, bring to a simmer and cook over heat for 17 minutes. Divide the mix between plates and serve.

Nutrition: calories 120, fat 8, fiber 1, carbs 3, protein 7

Sesame Savoy Cabbage

Everyone can make this simple keto dish! You'll see!

Preparation time: 5 minutes
Cooking time: 20 minutes
Servings: 4

Ingredients:
- 2 garlic cloves, minced
- 2 spring onions, chopped
- 1 Savoy cabbage, shredded
- 1 tablespoon olive oil
- ½ cup tomato passata
- 1 tablespoon sesame seeds

Directions:
Heat up a pan with the oil over medium heat, add the spring onions and the garlic and sauté for 5 minutes. Add the cabbage and the rest of the ingredients, toss, cook over medium heat for 15 minutes more, divide between plates and serve.

Nutrition: calories 120, fat 3, fiber 1, carbs 3, protein 6

Chili Collard Greens

This will really make everyone love your cooking!

Preparation time: 10 minutes
Cooking time: 20 minutes
Servings: 4

Ingredients:
- 1 tablespoon chili powder
- 1 bunch collard greens, roughly chopped
- 1 tablespoon olive oil
- ½ cup chicken stock
- 2 shallots, chopped
- 1 teaspoon hot paprika
- ½ teaspoon cumin, ground
- A pinch of salt and black pepper
- 1 tablespoon lime juice

Directions:
Heat up a pan with the oil over medium high heat, add the shallots and sauté for 5 minutes. Add the collard greens and the other ingredients, toss and cook over medium heat for 15 minutes more. Divide everything between plates and serve.

Nutrition: calories 245, fat 20, fiber 1, carbs 5, protein 12

Artichokes Soup

This is a keto soup even vegetarians will love!

Preparation time: 10 minutes
Cooking time: 35 minutes
Servings: 6

Ingredients:

- 1 tablespoon olive oil
- 2 shallots, chopped
- 10 ounces canned artichokes, drained and quartered
- 4 cups chicken stock
- 1 teaspoon smoked paprika
- 1 teaspoon cumin, ground
- A pinch of red pepper flakes
- 3 celery stalks, chopped
- 2 tomatoes, cubed
- 2 tablespoons lime juice
- A pinch of salt and black pepper

Directions:

Heat up a pot with the oil over medium high heat, add the shallots and sauté for 5 minutes. Add the artichokes and the other ingredients, bring to a simmer and cook over medium heat for 30 minutes more. Ladle the soup into bowls and serve.

Nutrition: calories 150, fat 3, fiber 2, carbs 4, protein 8

Ginger and Bok Choy Soup

This is a fresh spring Ketogenic soup!

Preparation time: 10 minutes
Cooking time: 25 minutes
Servings: 4

Ingredients:

- 4 cups bok choy, roughly chopped
- 2 spring onions, chopped
- 1 quart vegetable stock
- A pinch of salt and black pepper
- 2 teaspoons ginger, grated

Directions:

Put the stock into a pot, bring to a simmer over medium heat, add the bok choy and the other ingredients, bring to a simmer and cook for 25 minutes. Blend the soup using an immersion blender, divide into bowls and serve.

Nutrition: calories 140, fat 2, fiber 1, carbs 3, protein 7

Spinach Soup

This Indian style keto soup is amazing!

Preparation time: 10 minutes
Cooking time: 15 minutes
Servings: 4

Ingredients:

- 1 tablespoon olive oil
- ½ teaspoon coriander, ground
- 2 shallots, chopped
- 2 garlic cloves, minced
- 1 tablespoon ginger, grated
- 1 pound spinach leaves, torn
- 4 cups chicken stock
- A pinch of salt and black pepper
- 1 tablespoon cilantro, chopped

Directions:

Heat up a pot with the oil over medium high heat, add the shallots and the garlic and sauté for 2 minutes. Add the ginger, spinach and the other ingredients, bring to a simmer and cook over medium heat for 13 minutes more. Ladle the soup into bowls and serve.

Nutrition: calories 143, fat 6, fiber 3, carbs 7, protein 7

Asparagus Soup

It's incredibly easy and super delicious!

Preparation time: 10 minutes
Cooking time: 20 minutes
Servings: 4

Ingredients:

- 1 asparagus bunch, trimmed and halved
- 1 tablespoon olive oil
- 2 shallots, chopped
- 1 teaspoon lime juice
- 4 cups chicken stock
- 1 cup heavy cream
- A pinch of salt and black pepper
- 1 tablespoon oregano, chopped

Directions:

Heat up a pot with the oil over medium heat, add the shallots and sauté for 2 minutes. Add the asparagus and the other ingredients except the cream and the oregano, bring to a simmer and cook over medium heat for 18 minutes more. Add the cream, blend the soup using an immersion blender, divide into bowls and serve with the oregano sprinkled on top.

Nutrition: calories 130, fat 1, fiber 1, carbs 2, protein 3

Baked Endives

These will be ready in only 10 minutes!

Preparation time: 10 minutes
Cooking time: 20 minutes
Servings: 4

Ingredients:

- ¼ cup parmesan, grated
- 2 endives, trimmed and halved lengthwise
- 1 tablespoon olive oil
- 2 garlic cloves, minced
- A pinch of salt and black pepper
- ½ teaspoon sweet paprika

Directions:

Arrange the endives on a lined baking sheet, add the oil and the other ingredients, toss, introduce in the oven at 400 degrees F and bake for 20 minutes. Divide between plates and serve.

Nutrition: calories 120, fat 2, fiber 2, carbs 5, protein 8

Baked Asparagus

This keto dish is very delicious and it also looks wonderful!

Preparation time: 10 minutes
Cooking time: 15 minutes
Servings: 4

Ingredients:

- 1 tablespoon avocado oil
- 2 bunches of asparagus, trimmed
- 2 tablespoons lime juice
- ½ cup parmesan, grated
- A pinch of salt and black pepper

Directions:

Arrange the asparagus on a lined baking sheet, add the oil and the other ingredients, toss and bake at 400 degrees F for 15 minutes. Divide between plates and serve.

Nutrition: calories 160, fat 7, fiber 2, carbs 6, protein 10

Asparagus and Tomatoes

It's really, really tasty!

Preparation time: 10 minutes
Cooking time: 20 minutes
Servings: 4

Ingredients:

- ¼ cup shallots, chopped
- 2 tablespoons olive oil
- 4 asparagus spears, trimmed and halved
- 1 pound cherry tomatoes, halved
- A pinch of salt and black pepper
- 1 cup cheddar cheese, grated

Directions:

In a roasting pan, combine the asparagus with the shallots and the other ingredients, toss and bake at 400 degrees F for 20 minutes. Divide the mix between plates and serve.

Nutrition: calories 200, fat 12, fiber 2, carbs 5, protein 14

Endives and Mustard Sauce

It's a very creamy keto dish you can try tonight!

Preparation time: 10 minutes
Cooking time: 20 minutes
Servings: 4

Ingredients:

- 2 endives, trimmed and halved lengthwise
- 2 tablespoons olive oil
- 2 shallots, chopped
- A pinch of salt and black pepper
- 2 tablespoons parmesan, grated
- 2 tablespoons mustard
- ¼ cup heavy cream

Directions:

Heat up a pan with the oil over medium heat, add the shallots and sauté for 2 minutes. Add the endives and the other ingredients except the parmesan, toss, and cook over medium heat for 15 minutes more. Add the parmesan, toss, cook everything for 3 minutes more, divide between plates and serve.

Nutrition: calories 256, fat 23, fiber 2, carbs 5, protein 13

Baked Brussels Sprouts

This is so fresh and full of vitamins! It's wonderful!

Preparation time: 10 minutes
Cooking time: 20 minutes
Servings: 4

Ingredients:

- 1 pound Brussels sprouts, trimmed and halved
- 1 tablespoon avocado oil
- 2 garlic cloves, minced
- A pinch of salt and black pepper
- ¼ cup cilantro, chopped

Directions:

In a roasting pan, combine the sprouts with the oil and the other ingredients, toss and bake at 400 degrees F for 20 minutes. Divide everything between plates and serve.

Nutrition: calories 100, fat 3, fiber 1, carbs 2, protein 6

Roasted Tomatoes

If you don't have time to cook a complex dinner tonight, then try this!

Preparation time: 10 minutes
Cooking time: 25 minutes
Servings: 4

Ingredients:

- 1 pound tomatoes, halved
- A pinch of salt and black pepper
- 2 tablespoons olive oil
- 1 teaspoon rosemary, dried
- 1 teaspoon basil, dried
- 1 tablespoon chives, chopped

Directions:

In a roasting pan combine the tomatoes with the oil and the other ingredients, toss gently and bake at 390 degrees F for 25 minutes. Divide the mix between plates and serve.

Nutrition: calories 122, fat 12, fiber 1, carbs 3, protein 14

Brussels Sprouts and Green Beans
Do you want to learn how to make this tasty keto dish?.

Preparation time: 10 minutes
Cooking time: 20 minutes
Servings: 4

Ingredients:
- 1 tablespoon avocado oil
- 1 pound Brussels sprouts, trimmed and halved
- ½ pound green beans, trimmed and halved
- ½ teaspoon garlic powder
- A pinch of salt and black pepper
- 1 tablespoon lime juice

Directions:
In a roasting pan, combine the sprouts with the green beans and the other ingredients, toss, introduce in the oven at 375 degrees F and bake for 20 minutes. Divide between plates and serve.

Nutrition: calories 80, fat 5, fiber 2, carbs 5, protein 7

Crispy Radishes
It's a great keto idea!

Preparation time: 10 minutes
Cooking time: 20 minutes
Servings: 4

Ingredients:
- Cooking spray
- 15 radishes, sliced
- Salt and black pepper to the taste
- 1 tablespoon chives, chopped

Directions:
Arrange radish slices on a lined baking sheet and spray them with cooking oil.
Season with salt and pepper and sprinkle chives, introduce in the oven at 375 degrees F and bake for 10 minutes. Flip them and bake for 10 minutes more.
Serve them cold.

Nutrition: calories 30, fat 1, fiber 0.4, carbs 1, protein 0.1

Creamy Radishes
It's a creamy and tasty keto veggie dish!

Preparation time: 10 minutes
Cooking time: 25 minutes
Servings: 1

Ingredients:

- 7 ounces radishes, cut in halves
- 2 tablespoons sour cream
- 2 bacon slices
- 1 tablespoon green onion, chopped
- 1 tablespoon cheddar cheese, grated
- Hot sauce to the taste
- Salt and black pepper to the taste

Directions:

Put radishes into a pot, add water to cover, bring to a boil over medium heat, cook them for 10 minutes and drain. Heat up a pan over medium high heat, add bacon, cook until it's crispy, transfer to paper towels, drain grease, crumble and leave aside. Return pan to medium heat, add radishes, stir and sauté them for 7 minutes. Add onion, salt, pepper, hot sauce and sour cream, stir and cook for 7 minutes more. Transfer to a plate, top with crumbled bacon and cheddar cheese and serve.

Nutrition: calories 340, fat 23, fiber 3, carbs 6, protein 15

Radish Soup
Oh my God! This tastes divine!

Preparation time: 10 minutes
Cooking time: 20 minutes
Servings: 4

Ingredients:

- 2 bunches radishes, cut in quarters
- Salt and black pepper to the taste
- 6 cups chicken stock
- 2 stalks celery, chopped
- 3 tablespoons coconut oil
- 6 garlic cloves, minced
- 1 yellow onion, chopped

Directions:

Heat up a pot with the oil over medium heat, add onion, celery and garlic, stir and cook for 5 minutes. Add radishes, stock, salt and pepper, stir, bring to a boil, cover and simmer for 15 minutes. Divide into soup bowls and serve.

Nutrition: calories 120, fat 2, fiber 1, carbs 3, protein 10

Tasty Avocado Salad

This is very tasty and refreshing!

Preparation time: 10 minutes
Cooking time: 0 minutes
Servings: 4

Ingredients:
- 2 avocados, pitted and mashed
- Salt and black pepper to the taste
- ¼ teaspoon lemon stevia
- 1 tablespoon white vinegar
- 14 ounces coleslaw mix
- Juice from 2 limes
- ¼ cup red onion, chopped
- ¼ cup cilantro, chopped
- 2 tablespoons olive oil

Directions:
Put coleslaw mix in a salad bowl. Add avocado mash and onions and toss to coat. In a bowl, mix lime juice with salt, pepper, oil, vinegar and stevia and stir well. Add this over salad, toss to coat, sprinkle cilantro and serve.

Nutrition: calories 100, fat 10, fiber 2, carbs 5, protein 8

Avocado And Egg Salad

You will make it again for sure!

Preparation time: 10 minutes
Cooking time: 7 minutes
Servings: 4

Ingredients:
- 4 cups mixed lettuce leaves, torn
- 4 eggs
- 1 avocado, pitted and sliced
- ¼ cup mayonnaise
- 2 teaspoons mustard
- 2 garlic cloves, minced
- 1 tablespoon chives, chopped
- Salt and black pepper to the taste

Directions:
Put water in a pot, add some salt, add eggs, bring to a boil over medium high heat, boil for 7 minutes, drain, cool, peel and chop them. In a salad bowl, mix lettuce with eggs and avocado. Add chives and garlic, some salt and pepper and toss to coat. In a bowl, mix mustard with mayo, salt and pepper and stir well. Add this over salad, toss well and serve right away.

Nutrition: calories 234, fat 12, fiber 4, carbs 7, protein 12

Avocado And Cucumber Salad

You will ask for more! It's such a tasty summer salad!

Preparation time: 10 minutes
Cooking time: 0 minutes
Servings: 4

Ingredients:

- 1 small red onion, sliced
- 1 cucumber, sliced
- 2 avocados, pitted, peeled and chopped
- 1 pound cherry tomatoes, halved
- 2 tablespoons olive oil
- ¼ cup cilantro, chopped
- 2 tablespoons lemon juice
- Salt and black pepper to the taste

Directions:

In a large salad bowl, mix tomatoes with cucumber, onion and avocado and stir.
Add oil, salt, pepper and lemon juice and toss to coat well. Serve cold with cilantro on top.

Nutrition: calories 140, fat 4, fiber 2, carbs 4, protein 5

Delicious Avocado Soup

You will adore this special and delicious keto soup!

Preparation time: 10 minutes
Cooking time: 10 minutes
Servings: 4

Ingredients:

- 2 avocados, pitted, peeled and chopped
- 3 cups chicken stock
- 2 scallions, chopped
- Salt and black pepper to the taste
- 2 tablespoons ghee
- 2/3 cup heavy cream

Directions:

Heat up a pot with the ghee over medium heat, add scallions, stir and cook for 2 minutes. Add 2 and ½ cups stock, stir and simmer for 3 minutes. In your blender, mix avocados with the rest of the stock, salt, pepper and heavy cream and pulse well. Add this to the pot, stir well, cook for 2 minutes and season with more salt and pepper. Stir well, ladle into soup bowls and serve.

Nutrition: calories 332, fat 23, fiber 4, carbs 6, protein 6

Delicious Avocado And Bacon Soup

Have you ever heard about such a delicious keto soup? Then it's time you find out more about it!

Preparation time: 10 minutes
Cooking time: 10 minutes
Servings: 4

Ingredients:

- 2 avocados, pitted and cut in halves
- 4 cups chicken stock
- 1/3 cup cilantro, chopped
- Juice from ½ lime
- 1 teaspoon garlic powder
- ½ pound bacon, cooked and chopped
- Salt and black pepper to the taste

Directions:

Put stock in a pot and bring to a boil over medium high heat. In your blender, mix avocados with garlic powder, cilantro, lime juice, salt and pepper and blend well.
Add this over stock and blend using an immersion blender. Add bacon, more salt and pepper the taste, stir, cook for 3 minutes, ladle into soup bowls and serve.

Nutrition: calories 300, fat 23, fiber 5, carbs 6, protein 17

Thai Avocado Soup

This is a great and exotic soup!

Preparation time: 10 minutes
Cooking time: 10 minutes
Servings: 4

Ingredients:

- 1 cup coconut milk
- 2 teaspoons Thai green curry paste
- 1 avocado, pitted, peeled and chopped
- 1 tablespoon cilantro, chopped
- Salt and black pepper to the taste
- 2 cups veggie stock
- Lime wedges for serving

Directions:

In your blender, mix avocado with salt, pepper, curry paste and coconut milk and pulse well. Transfer this to a pot and heat up over medium heat. Add stock, stir, bring to a simmer and cook for 5 minutes. Add cilantro, more salt and pepper, stir, cook for 1 minute more, ladle into soup bowls and serve with lime wedges on the side.

Nutrition: calories 240, fat 4, fiber 2, carbs 6, protein 12

Simple Arugula Salad
It's light and very tasty! Try it for dinner!

Preparation time: 10 minutes
Cooking time: 0 minutes
Servings: 4

Ingredients:
- 1 white onion, chopped
- 1 tablespoon vinegar
- 1 cup hot water
- 1 bunch baby arugula
- ¼ cup walnuts, chopped
- 2 tablespoons cilantro, chopped
- 2 garlic cloves, minced
- 2 tablespoons olive oil
- Salt and black pepper to the taste
- 1 tablespoon lemon juice

Directions:
In a bowl, mix water with vinegar, add onion, leave aside for 5 minutes, drain well and press. In a salad bowl, mix arugula with walnuts and onion and stir. Add garlic, salt, pepper, lemon juice, cilantro and oil, toss well and serve.

Nutrition: calories 200, fat 2, fiber 1, carbs 5, protein 7

Arugula Soup
You have to try this great keto soup as soon as you can!

Preparation time: 10 minutes
Cooking time: 13 minutes
Servings: 6

Ingredients:
- 1 yellow onion, chopped
- 1 tablespoon olive oil
- 2 garlic cloves, minced
- ½ cup coconut milk
- 10 ounces baby arugula
- ¼ cup mixed mint, tarragon and parsley
- 2 tablespoons chives, chopped
- 4 tablespoons coconut milk yogurt
- 6 cups chicken stock
- Salt and black pepper to the taste

Directions:
Heat up a pot with the oil over medium high heat, add onion and garlic, stir and cook for 5 minutes. Add stock and milk, stir and bring to a simmer. Add arugula, tarragon, parsley and mint, stir and cook everything for 6 minutes. Add coconut yogurt, salt, pepper and chives, stir, cook for 2 minutes, divide into soup bowls and serve.

Nutrition: calories 200, fat 4, fiber 2, carbs 6, protein 10

Arugula And Broccoli Soup
It's one of out favorite soups!

Preparation time: 10 minutes
Cooking time: 20 minutes
Servings: 4

Ingredients:

- 1 small yellow onion, chopped
- 1 tablespoon olive oil
- 1 garlic clove, minced
- 1 broccoli head, florets separated
- Salt and black pepper to the taste
- 2 and ½ cups veggie stock
- 1 teaspoon cumin, ground
- Juice from ½ lemon
- 1 cup arugula leaves

Directions:

Heat up a pot with the oil over medium high heat, add onions, stir and cook for 4 minutes. Add garlic, stir and cook for 1 minute. Add broccoli, cumin, salt and pepper, stir and cook for 4 minutes. Add stock, stir and cook for 8 minutes. Blend soup using an immersion blender, add half of the arugula and blend again. Add the rest of the arugula, stir and heat up the soup again. Add lemon juice, stir, ladle into soup bowls and serve.

Nutrition: calories 150, fat 3, fiber 1, carbs 3, protein 7

Delicious Zucchini Cream
This is a keto comfort food you will enjoy for sure!

Preparation time: 10 minutes
Cooking time: 25 minutes
Servings: 8

Ingredients:

- 6 zucchinis, cut in halves, sliced
- Salt and black pepper to the taste
- 1 tablespoon ghee
- 28 ounces veggie stock
- 1 teaspoon oregano, dried
- ½ cup yellow onion, chopped
- 3 garlic cloves, minced
- 2 ounces parmesan, grated
- ¾ cup heavy cream

Directions:

Heat up a pot with the ghee over medium high heat, add onion, stir and cook for 4 minutes. Add garlic, stir and cook for 2 minutes more. Add zucchinis, stir and cook for 3 minutes. Add stock, stir, bring to a boil and simmer over medium heat for 15 minutes. Add oregano, salt and pepper, stir, take off heat and blend using an immersion blender. Heat up soup again, add heavy cream, stir and bring to a simmer. Add parmesan, stir, take off heat, ladle into bowls and serve right away.

Nutrition: calories 160, fat 4, fiber 2, carbs 4, protein 8

Zucchini And Avocado Soup

This keto soup is full of tasty ingredient and healthy elements!

Preparation time: 10 minutes
Cooking time: 15 minutes
Servings: 4
Ingredients:

- 1 big avocado, pitted, peeled and chopped
- 4 scallions, chopped
- 1 teaspoon ginger, grated
- 2 tablespoons avocado oil
- Salt and black pepper to the taste
- 2 zucchinis, chopped
- 29 ounces veggie stock
- 1 garlic clove, minced
- 1 cup water
- 1 tablespoon lemon juice
- 1 red bell pepper, chopped

Directions:

Heat up a pot with the oil over medium heat, add onions, stir and cook for 3 minutes. Add garlic and ginger, stir and cook for 1 minute. Add zucchini, salt, pepper, water and stock, stir, bring to a boil, cover pot and cook for 10 minutes. Take off heat, leave soup aside for a couple of minutes, add avocado, stir, blend everything using an immersion blender and heat up again. Add more salt and pepper, bell pepper and lemon juice, stir, heat up soup again, ladle into soup bowls and serve.

Nutrition: calories 154, fat 12, fiber 3, carbs 5, protein 4

Swiss Chard Pie

You will always remember this amazing taste!

Preparation time: 10 minutes
Cooking time: 45 minutes
Servings: 12
Ingredients:

- 8 cups Swiss chard, chopped
- ½ cup onion, chopped
- 1 tablespoon olive oil
- 1 garlic clove, minced
- Salt and black pepper to the taste
- 3 eggs
- 2 cups ricotta cheese
- 1 cup mozzarella, shredded
- A pinch of nutmeg
- ¼ cup parmesan, grated
- 1 pound sausage, chopped

Directions:

Heat up a pan with the oil over medium heat, add onions and garlic, stir and cook for 3 minutes. Add Swiss chard, stir and cook for 5 minutes more. Add salt, pepper and nutmeg, stir, take off heat and leave aside for a few minutes. In a bowl, whisk eggs with mozzarella, parmesan and ricotta and stir well. Add Swiss chard mix and stir well. Spread sausage meat on the bottom of a pie pan and press well. Add Swiss chard and eggs mix, spread well, introduce in the oven at 350 degrees F and bake for 35 minutes. Leave pie aside to cool down, slice and serve it.

Nutrition: calories 332, fat 23, fiber 3, carbs 4, protein 23

Swiss Chard Salad

This keto salad is perfect for a quick dinner!

Preparation time: 10 minutes
Cooking time: 20 minutes
Servings: 4

Ingredients:

- 1 bunch Swiss chard, cut in strips
- 2 tablespoons avocado oil
- 1 small yellow onion, chopped
- A pinch of red pepper flakes
- ¼ cup pine nuts, toasted
- ¼ cup raisins
- 1 tablespoon balsamic vinegar
- Salt and black pepper to the taste

Directions:

Heat up a pan with the oil over medium heat, add chard and onions, stir and cook for 5 minutes. Add salt, pepper and pepper flakes, stir and cook for 3 minutes more. Put raisins in a bowl, add water to cover them, heat them up in your microwave for 1 minute, leave aside for 5 minutes and drain them well. Add raisins and pine nuts to the pan, also add vinegar, stir, cook for 3 minutes more, divide on plates and serve.

Nutrition: calories 120, fat 2, fiber 1, carbs 4, protein 8

Green Salad

You must try this keto salad!

Preparation time: 10 minutes
Cooking time: 0 minutes
Servings: 4

Ingredients:

- 4 handfuls grapes, halved
- 1 bunch Swiss chard, chopped
- 1 avocado, pitted, peeled and cubed
- Salt and black pepper to the taste
- 2 tablespoons avocado oil
- 1 tablespoon mustard
- 7 sage leaves, chopped
- 1 garlic clove, minced

Directions:

In a salad bowl, mix Swiss chard with grapes and avocado cubes. In a bowl, mix mustard with oil, sage, garlic, salt and pepper and whisk well. Add this over salad, toss to coat well and serve.

Nutrition: calories 120, fat 2, fiber 1, carbs 4, protein 5

Catalan Style Greens
This veggie keto dish is just great!

Preparation time: 10 minutes
Cooking time: 15 minutes
Servings: 4

Ingredients:
- 1 apple, cored and chopped
- 1 yellow onion, sliced
- 3 tablespoons avocado oil
- ¼ cup raisins
- 6 garlic cloves, chopped
- ¼ cup pine nuts, toasted
- ¼ cup balsamic vinegar
- 5 cups mixed spinach and chard
- Salt and black pepper to the taste
- A pinch of nutmeg

Directions:
Heat up a pan with the oil over medium high heat, add onion, stir and cook for 3 minutes. Add apple, stir and cook for 4 minutes more. Add garlic, stir and cook for 1 minute. Add raisins, vinegar and mixed spinach and chard, stir and cook for 5 minutes. Add nutmeg, salt and pepper, stir, cook for a few seconds more, divide on plates and serve.

Nutrition: calories 120, fat 1, fiber 2, carbs 3, protein 6

Swiss Chard Soup
This is very hearth and rich!

Preparation time: 10 minutes
Cooking time: 35 minutes
Servings: 12
Ingredients:
- 4 cups Swiss chard, chopped
- 4 cups chicken breast, cooked
- 2 cups water
- 1 cup mushrooms, sliced
- 1 tablespoon garlic, minced
- 1 tablespoon coconut oil, melted
- ¼ cup onion, chopped
- 8 cups chicken stock
- 2 cups yellow squash, chopped
- 1 cup green beans
- 2 tablespoons vinegar
- ¼ cup basil, chopped
- 4 bacon slices, chopped
- ¼ cup sundried tomatoes

Directions:
Heat up a pot with the oil over medium high heat, add bacon, stir and cook for 2 minutes. Add tomatoes, garlic, onions and mushrooms, stir and cook for 5 minutes. Add water, stock and chicken, stir and cook for 15 minutes. Add Swiss chard, green beans, squash, salt and pepper, stir and cook for 10 minutes more.
Add vinegar, basil, more salt and pepper if needed, stir, ladle into soup bowls and serve.

Nutrition: calories 140, fat 4, fiber 2, carbs 4, protein 18

Special Swiss Chard Soup

His is so amazing!

Preparation time: 10 minutes
Cooking time: 2 hours and 10 minutes
Servings: 4
Ingredients:

- 1 red onion, chopped
- 1 bunch Swiss chard, chopped
- 1 yellow squash, chopped
- 1 zucchini, chopped
- 1 green bell pepper, chopped
- Salt and black pepper to the taste
- 6 carrots, chopped
- 4 cups tomatoes, chopped
- 1 cup cauliflower florets, chopped
- 1 cup green beans, chopped
- 6 cups chicken stock
- 7 ounces canned tomato paste
- 2 cups water
- 1 pound sausage, chopped
- 2 garlic cloves, minced
- 2 teaspoons thyme, chopped
- 1 teaspoon rosemary, dried
- 1 tablespoon fennel, minced
- ½ teaspoon red pepper flakes
- Some grated parmesan for serving

Directions:

Heat up a pan over medium high heat, add sausage and garlic, stir and cook until it browns and transfer along with its juices to your slow cooker. Add onion, Swiss chard, squash, bell pepper, zucchini, carrots, tomatoes, cauliflower, green beans, tomato paste, stock, water, thyme, fennel, rosemary, pepper flakes, salt and pepper, stir, cover and cook on High for 2 hours. Uncover pot, stir soup, ladle into bowls, sprinkle parmesan on top and serve.

Nutrition: calories 150, fat 8, fiber 2, carbs 4, protein 9

Roasted Tomato Cream

It will make your day a lot easier!

Preparation time: 10 minutes
Cooking time: 1 hour
Servings: 8

Ingredients:

1 jalapeno pepper, chopped
4 garlic cloves, minced
2 pounds cherry tomatoes, cut in halves
1 yellow onion, cut in wedges
Salt and black pepper to the taste
¼ cup olive oil
½ teaspoon oregano, dried
4 cups chicken stock
¼ cup basil, chopped
½ cup parmesan, grated

Directions:

Spread tomatoes and onion in a baking dish. Add garlic and chili pepper, season with salt, pepper and oregano and drizzle the oil. Toss to coat and bake in the oven at 425 degrees F for 30 minutes. Take tomatoes mix out of the oven, transfer to a pot, add stock and heat everything up over medium high heat. Bring to a boil, cover pot, reduce heat and simmer for 20 minutes. Blend using an immersion blender, add salt and pepper to the taste and basil, stir and ladle into soup bowls. Sprinkle parmesan on top and serve.

Nutrition: calories 140, fat 2, fiber 2, carbs 5, protein 8

Eggplant Soup

This is just what you needed today!

Preparation time: 10 minutes
Cooking time: 50 minutes
Servings: 4

Ingredients:

- 4 tomatoes
- 1 teaspoon garlic, minced
- ¼ yellow onion, chopped
- Salt and black pepper to the taste
- 2 cups chicken stock
- 1 bay leaf
- ½ cup heavy cream
- 2 tablespoons basil, chopped
- 4 tablespoons parmesan, grated
- 1 tablespoon olive oil
- 1 eggplant, chopped

Directions:

Spread eggplant pieces on a baking sheet, mix with oil, onion, garlic, salt and pepper, introduce in the oven at 400 degrees F and bake for 15 minutes. Put water in a pot, bring to a boil over medium heat, add tomatoes, steam them for 1 minutes, peel them and chop. Take eggplant mix out of the oven and transfer to a pot. Add tomatoes, stock, bay leaf, salt and pepper, stirz brin to a boil and simmer fro 30 minutes. Add heavy cream, basil and parmesan, stir, ladle into soup bowls and serve.

Nutrition: calories 180, fat 2, fiber 3, carbs 5, protein 10

Eggplant Stew

This is perfect for a family meal!

Preparation time: 10 minutes
Cooking time: 30 minutes
Servings: 4

Ingredients:

- 1 red onion, chopped
- 2 garlic cloves, chopped
- 1 bunch parsley, chopped
- Salt and black pepper to the taste
- 1 teaspoon oregano, dried
- 2 eggplants, cut in medium chunks
- 2 tablespoons olive oil
- 2 tablespoons capers, chopped
- 1 handful green olives, pitted and sliced
- 5 tomatoes, chopped
- 3 tablespoons herb vinegar

Directions:

Heat up a pot with the oil over medium heat, add eggplant, oregano, salt and pepper, stir and cook for 5 minutes. Add garlic, onion and parsley, stir and cook for 4 minutes. Add capers, olives, vinegar and tomatoes, stir and cook for 15 minutes. Add more salt and pepper if needed, stir, divide into bowls and serve.

Nutrition: calories 200, fat 13, fiber 3, carbs 5, protein 7

Roasted Bell Peppers Soup

This is not just very delicious! It's keto and healthy as well!

Preparation time: 10 minutes
Cooking time: 15 minutes
Servings: 6

Ingredients:
- 12 ounces roasted bell peppers, chopped
- 2 tablespoons olive oil
- 2 garlic cloves, minced
- 29 ounces canned chicken stock
- Salt and black pepper to the taste
- 7 ounces water
- 2/3 cup heavy cream
- 1 yellow onion, chopped
- ¼ cup parmesan, grated
- 2 celery stalks, chopped

Directions:
Heat up a pot with the oil over medium heat, add onion, garlic, celery, some salt and pepper, stir and cook for 8 minutes. Add bell peppers, water and stock, stir, bring to a boil, cover, reduce heat and simmer for 5 minutes. Use an immersion blender to puree the soup, then add more salt, pepper and cream, stir, bring to a boil and take off heat. Ladle into bowls, sprinkle parmesan and serve.

Nutrition: calories 176, fat 13, fiber 1, carbs 4, protein 6

Delicious Cabbage Soup

This delicious cabbage soup will become your new favorite keto soup really soon!

Preparation time: 10 minutes
Cooking time: 45 minutes
Servings: 8

Ingredients:
- 1 garlic clove, minced
- 1 cabbage head, chopped
- 2 pounds beef, ground
- 1 yellow onion, chopped
- 1 teaspoon cumin
- 4 bouillon cubes
- Salt and black pepper to the taste
- 10 ounces canned tomatoes and green chilies
- 4 cups water

Directions:
Heat up a pan over medium heat, add beef, stir and brown for a few minutes.
Add onion, stir, cook for 4 minutes more and transfer to a pot. Heat up, add cabbage, cumin, garlic, bouillon cubes, tomatoes and chilies and water, stir, bring to a boil over high heat, cover, reduce temperature and cook for 40 minutes. Season with salt and pepper, stir, ladle into soup bowls and serve.

Nutrition: calories 200, fat 3, fiber 2, carbs 6, protein 8

Ketogenic Dessert Recipes

Chocolate Pudding

These is so wonderful and delicious!

Preparation time: 10 minutes
Cooking time: 20 minutes
Servings: 4

Ingredients:

- 2 tablespoons cocoa powder
- 2 tablespoons ghee, melted
- 2/3 cup heavy cream
- 2 tablespoons swerve
- ¼ teaspoon vanilla extract

Directions:
In a bowl, combine the cocoa with the ghee and the other ingredients whisk well and divide into 4 ramekins. Bake at 350 degrees F for 20 minutes and serve warm.

Nutrition: calories 134, fat 14.1, fiber 0.8, carbs 3.1, protein 0.9

Coffee Cream

This looks and tastes wonderful!

Preparation time: 10 minutes
Cooking time: 15 minutes
Servings: 4

Ingredients:

- ¼ cup brewed coffee
- 2 tablespoons swerve
- 2 cups heavy cream
- 1 teaspoon vanilla extract
- 2 tablespoons ghee, melted
- 2 eggs

Directions:
In a bowl, mix the coffee with the cream and the other ingredients, whisk well and divide into 4 ramekins and whisk well. Introduce the ramekins in the oven at 350 degrees F and bake for 15 minutes. Serve warm.

Nutrition: calories 300, fat 30.8, fiber 0, carbs 3, protein 4

Walnut Balls

You must try these today!

Preparation time: 10 minutes
Cooking time: 0 minutes
Servings: 6
Ingredients:

- ½ cup ghee, melted
- 4 tablespoons walnuts, chopped
- 1 tablespoon stevia
- ¼ cup coconut flesh, unsweetened and shredded

Directions:

In a bowl, combine the walnuts with the ghee and the other ingredients, stir well and spoon into round moulds. Keep in the fridge until you serve them.

Nutrition: calories 194, fat 21.2, fiber 0.7, carbs 1, protein 1.4

Vanilla Cream

It's more than you can imagine!

Preparation time: 10 minutes
Cooking time: 20 minutes
Servings: 4
Ingredients:

- 2 cups heavy cream
- 2 tablespoons stevia
- 1 teaspoon vanilla extract
- 1 cup heavy cream
- 2 eggs, whisked
- 1 teaspoon baking powder

Directions:

In a bowl, combine the cream with the stevia and the other ingredients and whisk well. Divide into 4 ramekins, cook at 390 degrees F for 20 minutes, cool down and serve.

Nutrition: calories 346, fat 35.5, fiber 0, carbs 3.4, protein 4.6

Berry Cream

It's so delicious!

Preparation time: 10 minutes
Cooking time: 20 minutes
Servings: 4
Ingredients:

- 1 cup cream cheese
- 2 cups blackberries
- 1 tablespoon lime juice
- 1 tablespoon swerve
- ½ cup heavy cream

Directions:

In your blender, combine the blackberries with the cream and the other ingredients, pulse well and divide into 4 ramekins. Bake at 350 degrees F for 20 minutes, cool down and serve.

Nutrition: calories 289, fat 26.1, fiber 3.9, carbs 10.3, protein 5.7

Cream Cheese Ramekins

This special dessert will impress your loved ones for sure!

Preparation time: 10 minutes
Cooking time: 15 minutes
Servings: 6

Ingredients:

- 1 tablespoon vanilla extract
- 3 tablespoons ghee, melted
- 16 ounces cream cheese
- ½ cup swerve
- 1 teaspoon vanilla extract

Directions:

In a bowl, combine the vanilla with the ghee and the other ingredients, whisk well, divide into 6 ramekins, bake at 350 degrees F for 15 minutes, cool down and serve.

Nutrition: calories 329, fat 32.7, fiber 0, carbs 2.5, protein 5.7

Avocado Cream

This is a keto friendly dessert idea you must try!

Preparation time: 10 minutes
Cooking time: 15 minutes
Servings: 4

Ingredients:

- 2 tablespoons avocado oil
- 8 ounces cream cheese
- 2 avocados, peeled, pitted and mashed
- 2 eggs, whisked
- 1 teaspoon baking powder
- ½ cup swerve

Directions:

In your blender, combine the cream cheese with the avocados and the other ingredients, pulse well, divide into 4 ramekins and bake at 360 degrees F for 15 minutes. Cool the cream down and serve.

Nutrition: calories 312, fat 29.5, fiber 3.3, carbs 16.7, protein 8

Strawberry Stew

This is easy to make!

Preparation time: 10 minutes
Cooking time: 15 minutes
Servings: 4

Ingredients:
- ½ cup swerve
- 1 pound strawberries, halved
- 2 cups water
- 1 teaspoon vanilla extract

Directions:
In a pan, combine the strawberries with the swerve and the other ingredients, toss gently, bring to a simmer and cook over medium heat for 15 minutes. Divide into bowls and serve cold.

Nutrition: calories 40, fat 4.3, fiber 2.3, carbs 3.4, protein 0.8

Coconut Muffins

Everyone will adore these coconut delights!

Preparation time: 10 minutes
Cooking time: 25 minutes
Servings: 8

Ingredients:
- ½ cup ghee, melted
- 3 tablespoons swerve
- 1 cup coconut, unsweetened and shredded
- ¼ cup cocoa powder
- 2 eggs, whisked
- ¼ teaspoon vanilla extract
- 1 teaspoon baking powder

Directions:
In bowl, combine the ghee with the swerve, coconut and the other ingredients, stir well and divide into a lined muffin pan. Bake at 370 degrees F for 25 minutes, cool down and serve.

Nutrition: calories 344, fat 35.1, fiber 3.4, carbs 8.3, protein 4.5

Blueberries Mousse

This is just hypnotizing! It's great!

Preparation time: 10 minutes
Cooking time: 0 minutes
Servings: 6
Ingredients:

- 8 ounces heavy cream
- 1 teaspoon vanilla extract
- 1 tablespoon stevia
- 1 cup blueberries

Directions:

In a blender, combine the cream with the other ingredients, pulse well, divide into bowls and serve cold.

Nutrition: calories 219, fat 21.1, fiber 0.9, carbs 7, protein 1.4

Almond Berries Mix

You only need a few ingredients to make this!

Preparation time: 10 minutes
Cooking time: 12 minutes
Servings: 4
Ingredients:

- 1 cup almonds, chopped
- 1 cup strawberries
- 1 cup blackberries
- ¼ cup coconut milk
- 1 tablespoon stevia

Directions:

In a pan, combine the almonds with the strawberries and the other ingredients, bring to a simmer and cook over medium heat for 12 minutes. Divide the mix into bowls and serve.

Nutrition: calories 265, fat 6.3, fiber 2, carbs 4, protein 6

Lime and Watermelon Mousse

This is so refreshing and delicious!

Preparation time: 10 minutes
Cooking time: 0 minutes
Servings: 4
Ingredients:

- 1 cup heavy cream
- 1 tablespoon lime juice
- 1 tablespoon lime zest, grated
- 2 cups watermelon, peeled and cubed
- 1 cup cream cheese

Directions:

In a blender, combine the cream with the lime juice and the other ingredients, pulse well, divide into cups and serve cold.

Nutrition: calories 332, fat 31.4, fiber 0.5, carbs 9.2, protein 5.5

Eggs Cream

Try this cream on a summer day!

Preparation time: 2 hours
Cooking time: 10 minutes
Servings: 4

Ingredients:

- 4 eggs, whisked
- ¼ teaspoon vanilla extract
- ½ cup swerve
- 2 cups heavy cream
- ½ cup blackberries

Directions:

In a blender, combine the eggs with the vanilla and the other ingredients, pulse well, transfer to a pan, heat up over medium heat fro 10 minutes, divide into bowls, cool down and keep in the fridge for 2 hours before serving.

Nutrition: calories 243, fat 22, fiber 0, carbs 6.2, protein 4

Chia Squares

They look so good!

Preparation time: 10 minutes
Cooking time: 20 minutes
Servings: 6

Ingredients:

- 1 cup ghee, melted
- ½ teaspoon baking powder
- 3 tablespoons chia seeds
- 2 tablespoons swerve
- 1 cup cream cheese
- 6 eggs, whisked

Directions:

In a bowl, combine the ghee with the chia seeds and the other ingredients, whisk well, pour everything into a square baking dish, introduce in the oven at 350 degrees F and bake for 20 minutes. Cool down, slice into squares and serve.

Nutrition: calories 220, fat 2, fiber 0.5, carbs 2, protein 4

Plums Stew

This is simply excellent!

Preparation time: 10 minutes
Cooking time: 20 minutes
Servings: 4
Ingredients:

- 1 pound plums, pitted and halved
- 2 cups water
- 2 teaspoons vanilla
- 1 tablespoon lime juice
- 5 tablespoons swerve

Directions:

In a pan, combine the plums with the water and the other ingredients, bring to a simmer and cook over medium heat for 20 minutes. Divide the mix into bowls and serve.

Nutrition: calories 178, fat 4.4, fiber 2, carbs 3, protein 5

Plum Cream

This pudding is so tasty!

Preparation time: 30 minutes
Cooking time: 0 minutes
Servings: 4
Ingredients:

- 1 tablespoon swerve
- 1 cup plums, pitted, peeled
- 1 teaspoon vanilla extract
- 2 cups heavy cream

Directions:

In a blender, combine the plums with the swerve and the other ingredients, pulse well, divide into bowls and keep in the fridge for 30 minutes before serving.

Nutrition: calories 140, fat 2, fiber 2, carbs 4, protein 4

Cold Berries and Plums Bowls

These will make you fell amazing!

Preparation time: 5 minutes
Cooking time: 0 minutes
Servings: 4
Ingredients:

- 2 tablespoons swerve
- 1 cup plums, pitted and halved
- 1 teaspoon vanilla extract
- 1 cup blackberries
- 1 cup blueberries
- 2 tablespoons walnuts, chopped

Directions:

In a bowl, mix the plums with the blackberries and the other ingredients, toss and serve cold.

Nutrition: calories 400, fat 23, fiber 4, carbs 6, protein 7

Lime Avocado and Strawberries Mix

This is so easy to make at home and it follows keto principles!

Preparation time: 5 minutes
Cooking time: 0 minutes
Servings: 4

Ingredients:
- 2 avocados, pitted, peeled and cubed
- 1 cup strawberries, halved
- Juice of 1 lime
- 1 tablespoon stevia

Directions:
In a bow, combine the avocados with the strawberries, lime juice and stevia, toss and serve cold.

Nutrition: calories 150, fat 3, fiber 3, carbs 5, protein 6

Avocado and Watermelon Salad

It has such a fresh texture and taste!

Preparation time: 2 hours
Cooking time: 0 minutes
Servings: 4

Ingredients:
- 2 avocados pitted, peeled and cubed
- 2 cups watermelon, peeled and cubed
- 1 tablespoon stevia
- 1 cup heavy cream
- 1 tablespoon mint, chopped

Directions:
In a bowl, combine the avocados with the watermelon and the other ingredients, toss and keep in the fridge for 2 hours before serving.

Nutrition: calories 271, fat 24.5, fiber 6.3, carbs 14.1, protein 2.8

Coconut Raspberries Mix

You've got to love this keto mix!

Preparation time: 10 minutes
Cooking time: 15 minutes
Servings: 4

Ingredients:

- 1 cup coconut milk
- 2 tablespoons coconut flesh, unsweetened and shredded
- 1 cup raspberries
- 3 tablespoons swerve
- ½ teaspoon vanilla extract

Directions:

In a blender, combine the coconut with the raspberries and the other ingredients, pulse well, divide into 4 ramekins, introduce in the oven at 360 degrees F for 15 minutes, cool down and serve.

Nutrition: calories 393, fat 37.3, fiber 9.1, carbs 16.9, protein 4.2

Cinnamon Cream

You must try this special mix as well!

Preparation time: 2 hours
Cooking time: 10 minutes
Servings: 4

Ingredients:

- 2 tablespoons swerve
- 1 cup coconut milk
- 1 cup heavy cream
- 1 tablespoon cinnamon powder
- ¼ teaspoon ginger, ground

Directions:

In a bowl, combine the cream with the milk and the other ingredients, whisk well, transfer to a pot, heat up over medium heat for 10 minutes and divide into bowls.
Keep in the fridge for 2 hours before serving.

Nutrition: calories 244, fat 25.4, fiber 1.3, carbs 5.2, protein 2

Chocolate Cookies

This is an easy keto dessert idea!

Preparation time: 10 minutes
Cooking time: 20 minutes
Servings: 6
Ingredients:

- 2 cups walnuts, chopped
- 2 eggs, whisked
- ¼ cup avocado oil
- 2 tablespoons swerve
- ¼ cup cocoa powder
- 1 teaspoon baking powder

Directions:

In your food processor, combine the walnuts with the eggs and the other ingredients, pulse well, scoop tablespoons out of this mix, put them on a lined baking sheet, flatten them a bit and cook at 360 degrees F for 20 minutes.
Serve the cookies cold.
Nutrition: calories 452, fat 41.6, fiber 6.5, carbs 11.7, protein 19

Special Dessert

Have you tried this mix before?

Preparation time: 10 minutes
Cooking time: 0 minutes
Servings: 6
Ingredients:

- 1 cup blueberries
- 1 cup almonds, chopped
- ½ cup walnuts, chopped
- 1 cup blackberries
- 1 tablespoon swerve
- 1 tablespoon coconut oil, melted

Directions:

In a bowl, combine the berries with the almonds, and the other ingredients, toss and serve cold.
Nutrition: calories 223, fat 32, fiber 1, carbs 3, protein 6

Coconut and Mint Cookies

Serve this keto dessert right away!

Preparation time: 10 minutes
Cooking time: 15 minutes
Servings: 6
Ingredients:

- 1 cup almond flour
- 1 cup coconut, unsweetened and shredded
- 2 eggs, whisked
- ½ cup coconut cream
- ½ cup coconut oil, melted
- 3 tablespoons swerve
- 2 teaspoons mint, dried
- 2 teaspoons baking powder

Directions:

In a bowl, mix the almond flour with the coconut and the other ingredients, and stir well. Shape balls out of this mix, place them on a lined baking sheet, flatten them, introduce in the oven at 370 degrees F and bake for 15 minutes. Serve them cold.
Nutrition: calories 190, fat 7.32, fiber 2.2, carbs 4, protein 3

Avocado Bars

Even your kids will love this dessert!

Preparation time: 10 minutes
Cooking time: 30 minutes
Servings: 6

Ingredients:

- 1 teaspoon vanilla extract
- ½ cup ghee, melted
- 2 tablespoons swerve
- 1 avocado, peeled, pitted and mashed
- 2 cups almond flour
- 1 tablespoon cocoa powder

Directions:

In a bowl, mix the ghee with the vanilla and the other ingredients and stir everything. Transfer this to baking pan, spread evenly on the bottom, introduce in the oven at 350 degrees F and bake for 30 minutes. Cool down, cut into bars and serve.

Nutrition: calories 230, fat 12.2, fiber 4.2, carbs 5.4, protein 5.8

Orange Cake

You have to try this cake today!

Preparation time: 10 minutes
Cooking time: 20 minutes
Servings: 12

Ingredients:

- 6 eggs
- 1 orange, cut in quarters
- 1 teaspoon vanilla extract
- 1 teaspoon baking powder
- 9 ounces almond meal
- 4 tablespoons swerve
- A pinch of salt
- 2 tablespoons orange zest
- 2 ounces stevia
- 4 ounces cream cheese
- 4 ounces coconut yogurt

Directions:

In your food processor, pulse orange very well. Add almond meal, swerve, eggs, baking powder, vanilla extract and a pinch of salt and pulse well again. Transfer this into 2 spring form pans, introduce in the oven at 350 degrees F and bake for 20 minutes. Meanwhile, in a bowl, mix cream cheese with orange zest, coconut yogurt and stevia and stir well. Place one cake layer on a plate, add half of the cream cheese mix, add the other cake layer and top with the rest of the cream cheese mix. Spread it well, slice and serve.

Nutrition: calories 200, fat 13, fiber 2, carbs 5, protein 8

Tasty Nutella

Make your own keto nutella!

Preparation time: 10 minutes
Cooking time: 0 minutes
Servings: 6

Ingredients:
- 2 ounces coconut oil
- 4 tablespoons cocoa powder
- 1 teaspoon vanilla extract
- 1 cup walnuts, halved
- 4 tablespoons stevia

Directions:
In your food processor, mix cocoa powder with oil, vanilla, walnuts and stevia and blend very well. Keep in the fridge for a couple of hours and then serve.

Nutrition: calories 100, fat 10, fiber 1, carbs 3, protein 2

Mug Cake

This is very simple and tasty!

Preparation time: 2 minutes
Cooking time: 3 minutes
Servings: 1

Ingredients:
- 4 tablespoons almond meal
- 2 tablespoon ghee
- 1 teaspoon stevia
- 1 tablespoon cocoa powder, unsweetened
- 1 egg
- 1 tablespoon coconut flour
- ¼ teaspoon vanilla extract
- ½ teaspoon baking powder

Directions:
Put the ghee in a mug and introduce in the microwave for a couple of seconds. Add cocoa powder, stevia, egg, baking powder, vanilla and coconut flour and stir well. Add almond meal as well, stir again, introduce in the microwave and cook for 2 minutes. Serve your mug cake with berries on top.

Nutrition: calories 450, fat 34, fiber 7, carbs 10, protein 20

Delicious Sweet Buns

You will adore these keto buns and so will everyone else around you!

Preparation time: 10 minutes
Cooking time: 30 minutes
Servings: 8

Ingredients:
- ½ cup coconut flour
- 1/3 cup psyllium husks
- 2 tablespoons swerve
- 1 teaspoon baking powder
- A pinch of salt
- ½ teaspoon cinnamon
- ½ teaspoon cloves, ground
- 4 eggs
- Some chocolate chips, unsweetened
- 1 cup hot water

Directions:
In a bowl, mix flour with psyllium husks, swerve, baking powder, salt, cinnamon, cloves and chocolate chips and stir well. Add water and egg, stir well until you obtain a dough, shape 8 buns and arrange them on a lined baking sheet. Introduce in the oven at 350 degrees and bake for 30 minutes. Serve these buns with some almond milk and

Nutrition: calories 100, fat 3, fiber 3, carbs 6, protein 6

Lemon Custard

This is just irresistible!

Preparation time: 10 minutes
Cooking time: 30 minutes
Servings: 6

Ingredients:
- 1 and 1/3 pint almond milk
- 4 tablespoons lemon zest
- 4 eggs
- 5 tablespoons swerve
- 2 tablespoons lemon juice

Directions:
In a bowl, mix eggs with milk and swerve and stir very well. Add lemon zest and lemon juice, whisk well, pour into ramekins and place them into a baking dish with some water on the bottom. Bake in the oven at 360 degrees F for 30 minutes. Leave custard to cool down before serving it.

Nutrition: calories 120, fat 6, fiber 2, carbs 5, protein 7

Chocolate Ganache

It will be done in 5 minutes and it's completely Ketogenic!

Preparation time: 1 minute
Cooking time: 5 minutes
Servings: 6

Ingredients:

- ½ cup heavy cream
- 4 ounces dark chocolate

Directions:

Put cream into a pan and heat up over medium heat. Take off heat when it begins to simmer, add chocolate pieces and stir until it melts. Serve this very cold as a dessert or use it as a cream for a keto cake.

Nutrition: calories 78, fat 1, fiber 1, carbs 2, protein 0

Yummy Berries Dessert

You should try a new keto dessert each day! This is our suggestion for today!

Preparation time: 10 minutes
Cooking time: 0 minutes
Servings: 4

Ingredients:

- 3 tablespoons cocoa powder
- 14 ounces heavy cream
- 1 cup blackberries
- 1 cup raspberries
- 2 tablespoons stevia
- Some coconut chips

Directions:

In a bowl, whisk cocoa powder with stevia and heavy cream. Divide some of this mix into dessert bowls, add blackberries, raspberries and coconut chips, then spread another layer of cream and top with berries and chips. Serve these cold.

Nutrition: calories 245, fat 34, fiber 2, carbs 6, protein 2

Coconut Ice Cream

It's perfect for the summer!

Preparation time: 10 minutes
Cooking time: 0 minutes
Servings: 4

Ingredients:

- 1 mango, sliced
- 14 ounces coconut cream, frozen

Directions:

In your food processor, mix mango with the cream and pulse well. Divide into bowls and serve right away.

Nutrition: calories 150, fat 12, fiber 2, carbs 6, protein 1

Simple Macaroons

Try these keto macaroons and enjoy them!

Preparation time: 10 minutes
Cooking time: 10 minutes
Servings: 20

Ingredients:
- 2 tablespoons stevia
- 4 egg whites
- 2 cup coconut, shredded
- 1 teaspoon vanilla extract

Directions:
In a bowl, mix egg whites with stevia and beat using your mixer. Add coconut and vanilla extract and stir. Roll this mix into small balls and place them on a lined baking sheet. Introduce in the oven at 350 degrees F and bake for 10 minutes. Serve your macaroons cold.

Nutrition: calories 55, fat 6, fiber 1, carbs 2, protein 1

Simple Lime Cheesecake

It's the perfect cheesecake for a hot day!

Preparation time: 10 minutes
Cooking time: 2 minutes
Servings: 10

Ingredients:
- 2 tablespoons ghee, melted
- 2 teaspoons granulated stevia
- 4 ounces almond meal
- ¼ cup coconut, unsweetened and shredded
- *For the filling:*
- 1 pound cream cheese
- Zest from 1 lime
- Juice form 1 lime
- 2 sachets sugar free lime jelly
- 2 cup hot water

Directions:
Heat up a small pan over medium heat, add ghee and stir until it melts. In a bowl, mix coconut with almond meal, ghee and stevia and stir well. Press this on the bottom of a round pan and keep in the fridge for now. Meanwhile, put hot water in a bowl, add jelly sachets and stir until it dissolves. Put cream cheese in a bowl, add jelly and stir very well. Add lime juice and zest and blend using your mixer. Pour this over base, spread and keep the cheesecake in the fridge until you serve it.

Nutrition: calories 300, fat 23, fiber 2, carbs 5, protein 7

Coconut And Strawberry Delight

We won't tell you anything about this delight! Just pay attention!

Preparation time: 10 minutes
Cooking time: 0 minutes
Servings: 4

Ingredients:
- 1 and ¾ cups coconut cream
- 2 teaspoons granulated stevia
- 1 cup strawberries

Directions:
Put coconut cream in a bowl, add stevia and stir very well using an immersion blender. Add strawberries, fold them gently into the mix, divide dessert into glasses and serve them cold.

Nutrition: calories 245, fat 24, fiber 1, carbs 5, protein 4

Caramel Custard

It will be done in no time!

Preparation time: 10 minutes
Cooking time: 30 minutes
Servings: 2

Ingredients:
- 1 and ½ teaspoons caramel extract
- 1 cup water
- 2 ounces cream cheese
- 2 eggs
- 1 and ½ tablespoons swerve
- *For the caramel sauce:*
- 2 tablespoons swerve
- 2 tablespoons ghee
- ¼ teaspoon caramel extract

Directions:
In your blender, mix cream cheese with water, 1 and ½ tablespoons swerve, 1 and ½ teaspoons caramel extract and eggs and blend well. Pour this into 2 greased ramekins, introduce in the oven at 350 degrees F and bake for 30 minutes. Meanwhile, put the ghee in a pot and heat up over medium heat add ¼ teaspoon caramel extract and 2 tablespoons swerve, stir well and cook until everything melts. Pour this over caramel custard, leave everything to cool down and serve.

Nutrition: calories 254, fat 24, fiber 1, carbs 2, protein 8

Cookie Dough Balls

These are so amazing and delicious!

Preparation time: 10 minutes
Cooking time: 0 minutes
Servings: 10

Ingredients:
- ½ cup almond butter
- 3 tablespoons coconut flour
- 3 tablespoons coconut milk
- 1 teaspoon cinnamon, powder
- 3 tablespoons coconut sugar
- 15 drops vanilla stevia
- A pinch of salt
- ½ teaspoon vanilla extract
- *For the topping:*
- 1 and ½ teaspoon cinnamon powder
- 3 tablespoons granulated swerve

Directions:
In a bowl, mix almond butter with 1 teaspoon cinnamon, coconut flour, coconut milk, coconut sugar, vanilla extract, vanilla stevia and a pinch of salt and stir well.
Shape balls out of this mix. In another bowl mix 1 and ½ teaspoon cinnamon powder with swerve and stir well. Roll balls in cinnamon mix and keep them in the fridge until you serve.

Nutrition: calories 89, fat 1, fiber 2, carbs 4, protein 2

Ricotta Mousse

Serve this cold and

Preparation time: 2 hours and 10 minutes
Cooking time: 0 minutes
Servings: 10

Ingredients:
- ½ cup hot coffee
- 2 cups ricotta cheese
- 2 and ½ teaspoons gelatin
- 1 teaspoon vanilla extract
- 1 teaspoon espresso powder
- 1 teaspoon vanilla stevia
- A pinch of salt
- 1 cup whipping cream

Directions:
In a bowl, mix coffee with gelatin, stir well and leave aside until coffee is cold. In a bowl, mix espresso, stevia, salt, vanilla extract and ricotta and stir using a mixer. Add coffee mix and stir everything well. Add whipping cream and blend mixture again. Divide into dessert bowls and serve after you've kept it in the fridge for 2 hours.

Nutrition: calories 160, fat 13, fiber 0, carbs 2, protein 7

Dessert Granola

It's more than you could expect!

Preparation time: 10 minutes
Cooking time: 35 minutes
Servings: 4

Ingredients:

- 1 cup coconut, unsweetened and shredded
- 1 cup almonds and pecans, chopped
- 2 tablespoons stevia
- ½ cup pumpkin seeds
- ½ cup sunflower seeds
- 2 tablespoons coconut oil
- 1 teaspoon nutmeg, ground
- 1 teaspoon apple pie spice mix

Directions:

In a bowl, mix almonds and pecans with pumpkin seeds, sunflower seeds, coconut, nutmeg and apple pie spice mix and stir well. Heat up a pan with the coconut oil over medium heat, add stevia and stir until they combine. Pour this over nuts and coconut mix and stir well. Spread this on a lined baking sheet, introduce in the oven at 300 degrees F and bake for 30 minutes. Leave your granola to cool down, cut and serve it.

Nutrition: calories 120, fat 2, fiber 2, carbs 4, protein 7

Amazing Peanut Butter And Chia Pudding

The combination is very delicious!

Preparation time: 10 minutes
Cooking time: 0 minutes
Servings: 4

Ingredients:

- ½ cup chia seeds
- 2 cups almond milk, unsweetened
- 1 teaspoon vanilla extract
- ¼ cup peanut butter, unsweetened
- 1 teaspoon vanilla stevia
- A pinch of salt

Directions:

In a bowl, mix milk with chia seeds, peanut butter, vanilla extract, stevia and pinch of salt and stir well. Leave this pudding aside for 5 minutes, then stir it again, divide into dessert glasses and leave in the fridge for 10 minutes.

Nutrition: calories 120, fat 1, fiber 2, carbs 4, protein 2

Tasty Pumpkin Custard

It's one of our favorite keto desserts! Try it today!

Preparation time: 10 minutes
Cooking time: 5 minutes
Servings: 6

Ingredients:

- 1 tablespoon gelatin
- ¼ cup warm water
- 14 ounces canned coconut milk
- 14 ounces canned pumpkin puree
- A pinch of salt
- 2 teaspoons vanilla extract
- 1 teaspoon cinnamon powder
- 1 teaspoon pumpkin pie spice
- 8 scoops stevia
- 3 tablespoons erythritol

Directions:

In a pot, mix pumpkin puree with coconut milk, a pinch of salt, vanilla extract, cinnamon powder, stevia, erythritol and pumpkin pie spice, stir well and heat up for a couple of minutes. In a bowl, mix gelatin and water and stir. Combine the 2 mixtures, stir well, divide custard into ramekins and leave aside to cool down. Keep in the fridge until you serve it.

Nutrition: calories 200, fat 2, fiber 1, carbs 3, protein 5

No Bake Cookies

These are stunning and so yummy!

Preparation time: 40 minutes
Cooking time: 2 minutes
Servings: 4

Ingredients:

- 1 cup swerve
- ¼ cup coconut milk
- ¼ cup coconut oil
- 2 tablespoons cocoa powder
- 1 and ¾ cup coconut, shredded
- ½ teaspoon vanilla extract
- A pinch of salt
- ¾ cup almond butter

Directions:

Heat up a pan with the oil over medium high heat, add milk, cocoa powder and swerve, stir well for about 2 minutes and take off heat. Add vanilla, a pinch of salt, coconut and almond butter and stir very well. Place spoonfuls of this mix on a lined baking sheet, keep in the fridge for 30 minutes and then serve them.

Nutrition: calories 150, fat 2, fiber 1, carbs 3, protein 6

Butter Delight

It not just tasty! It also looks amazing!

Preparation time: 10 minutes
Cooking time: 4 minutes
Servings: 16

Ingredients:
- 4 ounces coconut butter
- 4 ounces cocoa butter
- ¼ cup swerve
- ½ cup peanut butter
- 4 ounces dark chocolate, sugar free
- ½ teaspoon vanilla extract
- 1/8 teaspoon xantham gum

Directions:
Put all butters and swerve in a pan and heat up over medium heat. Stir until they all combine and then mix with xantham gum and vanilla extract. Stir well again, pour into a lined baking sheet and spread well. Keep this in the fridge for 10 minutes. Heat up a pan with water over medium high heat and bring to a simmer. Add a bowl on top of the pan and add chocolate to the bowl. Stir until it melts and drizzle this over butter mix. Keep in the fridge until everything is firm, cut into 16 pieces and serve.

Nutrition: calories 176, fat 15, fiber 2, carbs 5, protein 3

Tasty Marshmallows

Did you know you can make the keto version at home?

Preparation time: 10 minutes
Cooking time: 3 minutes
Servings: 6

Ingredients:
- 2 tablespoons gelatin
- 12 scoops stevia
- ½ cup cold water
- ½ cup hot water
- 2 teaspoons vanilla extract
- ¾ cup erythritol

Directions:
In a bowl, mix gelatin with cold water, stir and leave aside for 5 minutes. Put hot water in a pan, add erythritol and stevia and stir well. Combine this with the gelatin mix, add vanilla extract and stir everything well. Beat this using a mixer and pour into a baking pan. Leave aside in the fridge until it sets, then cut into pieces and serve.

Nutrition: calories 140, fat 2, fiber 1, carbs 2, protein 4

Delicious Tiramisu Pudding

Try a keto tiramisu pudding today!

Preparation time: 2 hours and 10 minutes
Cooking time: 0 minutes
Servings: 1

Ingredients:

- 8 ounces cream cheese
- 16 ounces cottage cheese
- 2 tablespoons cocoa powder
- 1 teaspoon instant coffee
- 4 tablespoons almond milk
- 1 and ½ cup splenda

Directions:

In your food processor, mix cottage cheese with cream cheese, cocoa powder and coffee and blend very well.
Add splenda and almond milk, blend again and divide into dessert cups.
Keep in the fridge until you serve.

Nutrition: calories 200, fat 2, fiber 2, carbs 5, protein 5

Summer Dessert Smoothie

It's easy and super refreshing! You can try it today!

Preparation time: 5 minutes
Cooking time: 0 minutes
Servings: 2

Ingredients:

- ½ cup coconut milk
- 1 and ½ cup avocado, pitted and peeled
- 2 tablespoons green tea powder
- 2 teaspoons lime zest
- 1 tablespoon coconut sugar
- 1 mango thinly sliced for serving

Directions:

In your smoothie maker, combine milk with avocado, green tea powder and lime zest and pulse well. Add sugar, blend well, divide into 2 glasses and serve with mango slices on top.

Nutrition: calories 87, fat 5, fiber 3, carbs 6, protein 8

Lemon Sorbet

You only need 3 ingredients tom make this cool and keto dessert!

Preparation time: 5 minutes
Cooking time: 0 minutes
Servings: 4
Ingredients:

- 4 cups ice
- Stevia to the taste
- 1 lemon, peeled and roughly chopped

Directions:

In your blender, mix lemon piece with stevia and ice and blend until everything is combined.
Divide into glasses and serve very cold.

Nutrition: calories 67, fat 0, fiber 0, carbs 1, protein 1

Simple Raspberry Popsicles

It can't get any easier than this! You basically only need one ingredients: raspberries!

Preparation time: 2 hours
Cooking time: 10 minutes
Servings: 4
Ingredients:

- 1 and ½ cups raspberries
- 2 cups water

Directions:

Put raspberries and water in a pan, bring to a boil and simmer for 10 minutes at a medium temperature. Pour mix in an ice cube tray, stick popsicles sticks in each and chill in the freezer for 2 hours.

Nutrition: calories 60, fat 0, fiber 0, carbs 0, protein 2

Cherry And Chia Jam

Your family will love this great keto dessert!

Preparation time: 15 minutes
Cooking time: 12 minutes
Servings: 22
Ingredients:

- 3 tablespoons chia seeds
- 2 and ½ cups cherries, pitted
- ½ teaspoon vanilla powder
- Peel from ½ lemon, grated
- ¼ cup erythritol
- 10 drops stevia
- 1 cup water

Directions:

Put cherries and the water in a pot, add stevia, erythritol, vanilla powder, chia seeds and lemon peel, stir, bring to a simmer and cook for 12 minutes.
Take off heat and leave your jam aside for 15 minutes at least.
Serve cold.

Nutrition: calories 60, fat 1, fiber 1, carbs 2, protein 0.5

Conclusion

This is really a life changing cookbook. It shows you everything you need to know about the Ketogenic diet and it helps you get started.
You now know some of the best and most popular Ketogenic recipes in the world.
We have something for everyone's taste!

So, don't hesitate too much and start your new life as a follower of the Ketogenic diet! Get your hands on this special recipes collection and start cooking in this new, exciting and healthy way!

Have a lot of fun and enjoy your Ketogenic diet!

Printed in Great Britain
by Amazon